Praise for My Hungry Head

"*My Hungry Head* helped me believe there will always be food. I *knew* it, now I *believe* it. Now I can push the plate away." – Judi L.

"It's a process for me and my family. Our whole lives have changed, the way we shop, the way we eat, the way we interact with one another." – Emma S.

"I went to every class Marybeth had to offer. Her programs gave me connection and belonging. It's important to realize you're not alone – somehow sharing our experiences helped me move forward and find success with *My Hungry Head*." – Betty-Jo T.

The information in this book is creating and fortifying a movement towards a clearer, more actionable understanding of the mind/body connection. It's shifting the paradigm for all of us – from weight centric to body composition centric – and from just "healthy" eating to eating that's right for our individual needs. Indeed, it is a journey, but one well worth traveling. – Melody Marden, MS, CMCM

"Every weight-loss program needs a *My Hungry Head*. We can't help people lose weight without helping them keep it off." – Christine Labrecque, BSN, RN, CBN, Program Director

"This program is the perfect start on the journey to making peace with your weight and relationship with food." – Dr. Anita Johnson, best-selling author of *Eating by the Light of the Moon* and co-creator of Lightofthemooncafe.com

"Marybeth has created a road map for long-term success for all weight-loss patients." – Michael E. Jiser, MD

My Hungry Head

My Hungry Head

DISMANTLING THE DIET PRISON: A REAL LIFE GUIDE TO UNDERSTANDING YOUR BODY, CONTROLLING YOUR HUNGER AND TAKING CHARGE OF YOUR WEIGHT

Marybeth Sherrin

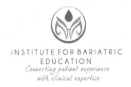

INSTITUTE FOR BARIATRIC
EDUCATION
*Connecting patient experience
with clinical expertise*

The information in this book is not intended to take the place of medical advice from a
trained medical professional who knows your detailed medical history. Every person has
unique medical issues that should be known to his or her medical provider. Readers are
advised to consult a physician or other qualified health professional regarding treatment
of any medical condition.

The names and other personal details of patient/participant stories in the text have been
changed to protect their privacy.

The trademark My Hungry Head® is registered in the U.S. Patent and Trademark Office.

For permission request or ordering information: Special discounts are available on
quantity purchases by hospitals, clinics, corporations, associations and others. For orders
by U.S. trade bookstores and wholesalers, please contact the Institute for Bariatric
Education LLC at 800-815-1344, or visit www.myhungryhead.com.

ISBN-13: 9780692704820 (My Hungry Head)

ISBN-10: 0692704825

Printed in the United States of America

To my father, "Big Bill," who battled obesity his entire life.
If only I could turn back time to ease your struggle.

Contents

Acknowledgements

I want to thank Maria Skinner for being an amazing partner, mentor and friend. She was the undeniable force behind this project. Special thanks to Paul Jablow for his skillful guidance and direction in helping us to share our expertise and tell our stories. Juli Warren, thank you for your proficient and efficient editing. And Paige Wojcukiewicz – wow – you have a fresh artistic voice and a superb ability to read my mind. Thanks for a super-fun cover.

McLean and Owen, you are my motivation. But I am overwhelmingly grateful to my husband, Alex. You are the quiet backbone of all I do. I can't imagine this adventure without you. To all of my family, especially my mom, Peg, Cath, Anna and Billy, thank you, thank you. It really takes a village.

Christine Labrecque, the last decade has been amazing. Thank you for always believing in my work and allowing me to make a difference. My deep appreciation to the surgeons and staff at Lowell General Hospital Center for Weight Management & Bariatric Surgery for all they do.

Lastly, I want to extend much love to the thousands of patients who have entrusted me with their stories – you have taught me the way. And to those who have shaped My Hungry Head as participants and shared your souls in our workshops and retreats, it truly has been a privilege to be part of *your* journey.

Marybeth Sherrin
May 2016

Foreword

I met Marybeth Sherrin in 2008 when she dropped into my dance class by mistake. She had meant to go to yoga, but found herself dancing – and liked it. Since 1997, I've been practicing and teaching movement techniques that invite participants to connect to their bodies, to seek pleasure in their movement, and to love their bodies – no matter what.

After a few classes, Marybeth was hooked. Then she was full of questions, and there our conversation – one that we are still having eight years later – began.

I became fascinated with her work as a behavioral therapist with surgical and non-surgical weight-loss patients. We began talking about how even after her patients have lost a tremendous amount of weight, many still did not feel good about themselves. Their bodies had changed, but their minds had not. Marybeth was also interested in offering movement options that made sense for her patients' physical shapes and fitness levels. She invited me to test a class or two at her clinic on Monday nights. This class is still running today – the clinic's longest-running movement program.

I never envisioned working with people struggling with obesity. They are not the usual attendees in my studio. But it didn't take long for me to fall in love with working with these patients. Many times, after they took their first class, they would say things like, "That is the first time I have ever felt beautiful" and "I didn't know I could move that way." I began getting to know those who came to class, and I listened to their stories. I heard about their experiences with their bodies, impending weight-loss surgery, or the way the surgery or their nutrition programs had gone for them. I heard the stories they tell themselves about who they are and how they look. And I heard what they can do now that they couldn't do while they were heavy.

In my classes, the invitation has always been to move in a way that feels good and to enjoy their bodies, a very new concept for many attendees. There is no judgment, which is something students clearly appreciate. As a teacher, I lead them, but I am also with them, part of their community. I witnessed how the strong connections they had to each other and their weight loss program were instrumental in their successes.

I began hearing about Marybeth's My Hungry Head class from the patients before Marybeth told me about it. They loved the My Hungry Head program, and they recommended it to other students who had not taken it. Once I learned more about it, the simplicity and the elegance of the program blew me away. On a personal level, I thought I had dealt with my own relationship with eating, but as I delved deeper into My Hungry Head, I realized that what I defined as "dealing" was still a Band-Aid of sorts. I was still spending too much of my precious life worrying about weight!

I was born in Montevideo, Uruguay, and lived there until I was 8 years old. We ate candy twice a year, during Christmas and Easter, as a special treat.

I loved to eat, and family celebrations centered on eating. My grandparents were all from Italy, where they had been mostly farmers and everybody had chickens, a backyard garden and fresh food. We loved to eat, but most of us were of average weight. I had one uncle who was very big – he was called Tio Gordo – "fat uncle." It was an affectionate term, but I also saw how it slowed him down.

In 1973, we moved to the United States. We left behind our extended family and the lifestyle of mostly homemade, fresh food. Across the street from our apartment building in Queens, New York, was a supermarket called Foodtown. We never saw so much food – we didn't know what hit us! We began eating prepared foods, and sugar became an everyday experience. Within a year, my 8-year-old mouth with no cavities in it had to get six fillings and surgery for gingivitis! My sisters, too, suddenly had mouths full of cavities. This is also when we, as a family, began struggling with weight.

My mom and her friends were always trying out new diets. I went on my first diet in middle school, to lose a "few pounds," and that began my own yoyo journey. Food was now something to be controlled and feared. This is about the time I began feeling imprisoned by food rather than enjoying it. My dad, on the other hand, was struggling with misdiagnosed diverticulitis. His doctor recommended a low-carb diet for him. This brought a lot of awareness into our house about food and gut issues. I was determined not to get fat and not to get sick.

I was always a mover and an explorer of ways to be healthy. My love of dance is what eventually made me realize that there were foods and substances that were addictive for me and that the choice of what to feed my body was mine. I had to change my eating habits, my mental attitude, and my feelings about my body, specifically around self-love. This all led me to where I am today, teaching people how to be in their bodies, how to eat in a way that helps them to thrive, and how to find their way – their own north. I can share my journey, but I know that everyone must make their own. There are no magic bullets, but there are ways in which we can support each other to live healthy, productive and passionate lives.

What I have seen at the clinic, in our retreats and in the community that Marybeth has developed around My Hungry Head is just such a support system. I have seen people come into the program, connect to each other, and transform their bodies, their minds and their lives. I am thrilled to have this program available to more people via this book and the My Hungry Head online educational program and live transformative retreats.

In tandem with Marybeth, I am committed to developing movement and personal exploration programs and projects including Move My Way™ and Imagine My Body™ to help men and women struggling with weight reimagine their relationship with themselves and their bodies in a way that is personal and truly empowering. This journey is all about freedom for me, and I feel so grateful to be surrounded by others who are living for the same.

Maria Skinner
www.huffingtonpost.com/maria-skinner

CHAPTER 1

Introduction

The secret of getting ahead is getting started.

– MARK TWAIN

B eth N. was able to "step away from food," stop binge eating and stabilize her weight after several years of consistent weight gain.

After undergoing gastric bypass surgery and "conquering my little inner critic," Patricia P. has gone from 262 pounds to 178. And stayed there.

Mike L. lost almost 100 pounds before weight-loss surgery and 190 more afterward. And he's keeping it off.

Brenda B., once afraid to do any group athletic activity, now goes ziplining and canoeing.

All four of these people have mastered the skill of lifetime weight control through the My Hungry Head program. We'll learn more about them and others like them in stories from the front lines of weight management.

For more than a decade, I've used this method to help hundreds of people develop a relationship with food that works for them and suits the way they live their lives – and keeps them at a stable weight.

Some of these people have gone through bariatric surgery, and some have not. What most of them have in common is that they have been what I call "serial dieters." They bounced from one fad diet to another, beating themselves up because nothing worked for more than a short while.

What they also had in common was expecting too much too soon. There is no magic bullet here. Weight control is a skill.

We've all had to master certain skills, whether it's learning to read as a child or learning what we need to know to do our jobs. This is no different. Which means you can do it.

One size does not fit all. Your body type, your metabolism, the demands of your daily routine – all influence what you need to do to reach a healthy weight and stay there. We are here to help you figure out what you need to succeed.

Losing weight and keeping it off is a complex process. It's more than just eating less and exercising more. Genetic, environmental, social and emotional factors play key roles in determining whether you lose weight and keep it off.

Learning how these factors affect you will take time and close observation. What won't help is guilt or shame. Shedding those can help you shed pounds. And you actually might find the experience enjoyable!

My Story

I'm Marybeth and I will be guiding you through your My Hungry Head journey. This program is very special to me, not only because I developed it, or because I love teaching it, or because my patients love following it. It's because it's changed me – and changed my life.

I've been a binge eater most of my life. And I got away with it for years. Until I couldn't.

Most of my life I was really skinny. I could eat anything I wanted and as much as I wanted, and I did. I amazed everyone with the amount of food I could get into my little body. Bingeing wasn't a problem for me. It was fun. Yet it was still bingeing.

In college, some kids binged on alcohol or played drinking games. Not me – I would be the one eating the sleeve of mint cookies or three cheeseburgers. I wasn't much of an athlete, but if there had been a competition for eating, I would have been an Olympian.

From a genetic perspective, I had hit the jackpot. I was born to a very fit and skinny mom and a morbidly obese dad, and I took after Mom.

But skinny genes only took me so far. As I got older, I got hooked into the diet trap and things began to change.

In my 20s, I hung out with athletes, primarily runners, who were obsessed with their weight. It was the late '80s and the fat-free craze was in full force. A popular book then was called *Eat to Win*. So I decided that I, too, needed to be on a diet if I wanted to "win." My carefree relationship with food became controlled, and suddenly my hunger felt like my worst enemy.

I read about tennis star Martina Navratilova's adherence to the Eat to Win diet and how, for example, she would eat pizza with the cheese scraped off and I figured that was for me.

I filled myself with carbs while conveniently ignoring the fact that she had a completely different body type and probably burned off more calories in an hour of practice than I did in a full day. I was also ignorant of how carbs affect hunger response. I was following somebody else's way.

No matter. I was off on the diet roller coaster, a ride that would last for years. The Atkins Diet. Low-calorie shake diet. The Cookie Diet. You name it, I tried it. The diet roller coaster, it seemed, was becoming my prison.

Like most people who diet, I could lose weight. I would lose a little water weight, a little fat, and little lean muscle each time I went on a diet.

At first, I was just trying to lose the 10 pounds that all the magazines said I should lose. Instead, I was putting on five pounds here, five pounds there. And then I would go back to my old ways. After all, who actually stays on a diet? Little did I know that every time I went on and off a diet, I was actually chipping away at my once-speedy metabolism. After every diet attempt, it would take more time and be a little harder to lose weight. Bye-bye, calorie-burning muscle. Hello, rebound pounds.

To make matters worse, every rise and dip in the roller coaster brought not just extra weight, but also a big dose of guilt and a feeling that I was just not disciplined enough. Instead of losing weight, I was losing self-esteem. This not only messed with my body, but also with my head.

Fast-forward a decade or two, and there I was – on the heavy end of the BMI chart! But in my mind, I was still the skinny little girl who could eat anything and everything. Binge eating was an automatic behavior. It was part of me.

Often, I would end an exhausting day at work with a trip through a McDonald's drive-through. I'd scarf down a burger and an apple pie and throw the wrappers out before going home to my husband and a full dinner. But of course I knew something was very wrong. I thought, I'm smart and I'm educated. I have a great career. Why can't I get this diet thing right? What's wrong with *me*?

With that question, I began the journey that brought me to My Hungry Head.

I was working primarily as a psychotherapist, but when an old colleague asked me to help out at a surgical weight-loss center, I started asking myself the questions that I would later teach my own patients to ask.

I dove into the patients' struggles. I was helping them prepare for surgery and adjust to life after weight loss. And at the same time, I began realizing that I had never developed the skill to take care of myself nutritionally.

I began to question not only the methods and diets I had been using, but also the state of mind created by the yoyo-ing.

Although I realized that restricting myself often led me right back to bingeing, I also realized that certain kinds of food made it much more difficult for me to stay on track and feel free in my mind.

I decided to replace the concept of "dieting" with new ways of thinking about eating. I began asking myself these two questions, not only as they pertained to food, but also as they pertained to everything in my life.

Does eating (doing) this make me feel out of control?
Does eating (doing) this make me feel bad (or sick)?

Over time, I have refined these questions. I have gone from eliminating foods that made me unable to stop myself from eating the whole thing to noticing subtle ways in which certain foods trigger cravings that I can choose to act on, or not act on, without feeling guilty or deprived. We will explore this more in the section about trigger foods.

"Sick" used to mean feeling really sick – nauseous or bloated or crampy. Now "sick" has a more refined meaning to me. It can be feeling discomfort as a result of what I ate or having headaches or dizziness from skipping meals. It can be a lethargic feeling after a meal when I felt energized before I ate.

This refinement has come as I've gotten to know myself and my body better. Once I was able to stabilize my eating patterns, I learned to listen to the quiet rhythms of my hunger cycle instead of my annoying, child-like voice crying for French fries and cake.

My journey hasn't been a perfect one, but once I accepted that being imperfect is OK, my travels became easier. There's a peacefulness in knowing that I don't always have to do this "right." Success is about creating the right circumstances so I do what's right for me.

Although I do not "diet," there are foods that I avoid. If something I eat makes me feel out of control or makes me sick, I am not going near it.

In the reference section, I will point you toward resources to help guide you on your journey, but most of all, I invite you to begin listening to yourself.

In the next chapters, we will explore internal and external factors that influence why, when, and how we eat. Some are biological, some are practical, and some are emotional.

You'll learn some of the key factors influencing your biological appetite so that you can reclaim what works for you and get to your own version of happy, healthy, and free. And free from your diet prison.

We All Have a Story

I can't recall one specific day or event when I realized I was a binger. Nor was there a specific day or event when I realized I was fixed. It was a process – and still is. Writing my story was the first step in this process.

Stories can be all sorts of things. Funny. Scary. Exciting. True. Fake. Distorted. Writing my story was scary and invigorating at the same time. The writing process itself helped me understand a lot about my eating and the way I learned, or didn't learn, to care for myself.

This week, take some time to write YOUR story. You don't have to share it if you don't want to. It's YOUR story to develop and understand. You decide what you want to do with it.

Go easy on yourself – approach this task like a screenwriter or playwright whose job is to write an amazing story of difficulties, challenges and triumph. Find yourself a quiet place and write your answers to the following questions:

How did your relationship with food develop?

_____

_____

_____

_____

_____

_____

_____

What stories do you tell yourself about eating, dieting, and weight as a child?

_____

_____

_____

_____

_____

_____

_____

As an adolescent?

_____

_____

_____

_____

_____

_____

As an adult?

_____

_____

_____

_____

_____

_____

How do you react when you have to "diet"?

_____

_____

_____

_____

_____

_____

When it comes to taking care of yourself, what's your greatest strength? (Yes, you must answer this!)

What's your greatest challenge in taking care of yourself?

_____

_____

_____

_____

_____

_____

_____

What are you hoping to change, shift, or improve as a result of the time you'll invest in the My Hungry Head process?

_____

_____

_____

_____

_____

_____

CHAPTER 2

Getting Started

*One of life's most painful moments comes
when we must admit that we didn't do our
homework, that we are not prepared.*

– Merlin Olsen

Of the thousands of patients that I've seen over the last decade, I assure you of this: I would be hard-pressed to find a single one who had set a goal to become obese. Not all my patients binge. And not all my patients eat until they're Thanksgiving-full. And no – they are not lazy. Most of my patients are hard-working, intelligent, creative people.

They come to My Hungry Head because they're searching for something that no commercial program or fad diet could provide.

This is what they tell me:

I want to be able to live without obsessing about food.
I want to eat to live, not live to eat.
I want to live long enough to see my kids get married.
I want to ride a bike.
I don't want to be turned away from an amusement park ride because I don't fit.
I want to be a role model for my kids.
I don't want to be out of breath anymore.

I don't want my weight to stop me from participating in life anymore.
I don't want to hear that I have a pretty face and I should just lose
some weight.
I want to feel good in my body. I want to like myself.

Many come to My Hungry Head feeling tired, defeated and disempowered. They are convinced that their doctors will have the "right" answer. Or that weight-loss surgery will finally prevent cravings and restore order between their brains and their stomachs. Most arrive to my class after the disappointing reality sets in – often months after surgery – or shortly after they've "hit goal" – that their body has changed, but their mind has not.

Remember: Surgeons can help you get the weight off, but only you can keep it off. After attending My Hungry Head, one patient referred to the workshop as bariatric brain surgery!

So what is it that we do? And how can you get started?

My Hungry Head is a big-girl, big-boy program – and I don't mean you have to weigh a lot to attend.

Think about this: If you've been on some kind of diet for half your life, like most of my patients, you have probably spent years and years being told what you should eat and how much you should move. And where did that get you?

After hearing hundreds of stories, I learned that most people with eating challenges may be generally nice on the outside, but they've become tough as nails on the inside. Initially, you can't see it. But if you look hard enough, you can see a giant middle finger, flipping off every diet coach that has crossed their path.

There's a good reason for this. The diet game is filled with one-size-fits-all solutions in which the dieter has no say. Individual needs and differences are irrelevant. Each diet is its own prison, in that it keeps you toggling between being "good" or being "bad," based on how well you are sticking to the diet. Yet who knows whether this is the right way for your body, your temperament and your taste? Look at it this way: If custom-tailored clothes were no more expensive than ready-made garments, who would ever buy off the rack?

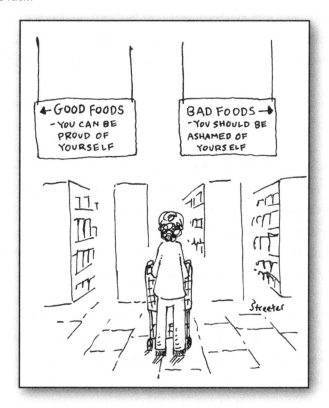

Honesty

OK, so how do we get started?

First we have to get honest. Magical and child-like thinking supports the billion-dollar diet industry – a desperate belief that there's a permanent cure to weight struggles. Now, not everyone sits in my office and says, "I want this program to make me lose weight and keep it off – forever." Well, actually, many say this – but it's followed up with: "I know these are just tools to help me" and "I know I'll have to work hard" and "I'm ready this time."

BUT ... 10, 12, 18 months after weight loss, cravings return, food is sexy again, the novelty has worn off. And frustration, disappointment and despair set in. Because let's face it, we really do want a magic cure – and that's OK.

What's not OK is to stay stuck in the endless search for the diet-pixie dust.

Honesty is our first tool. If you want to be successful at managing your weight, you've got to get honest. Not with me. With **yourself**. We'll question our beliefs about dieting. And we'll question the value of our family stories about eating and moving. We'll also question the overt and covert stories that we're told by marketing giants and media moguls. And more important, we'll question and explore what's best for ourselves.

I know, we've all manipulated our food journals. And we've all taken credit for more exercise than we really did. I mean, who hasn't shaken their Fitbit to get a few more steps in? And on some level, who hasn't bought into nonsense like this:

"If it is good for me, I can eat a lot of it."
"Calories don't count if I am just tasting something."
"I only ate the broken cookies."
"Food eaten on planes or in cars doesn't count."
"There are no calories if no one saw me eat it."

Don't worry, you're not alone!

But if we want real, lasting change, we have to start with the facts.

Take a few moments to honestly answer these questions. Start your journey by identifying what you're good at and what you will need to focus on. Answer each question based on where you are right now, NOT where you want to be.

1. Are you able to weigh yourself without negatively affecting your mood?

2. Do you make honest entries in a food or activity journal to learn how to improve your diet and lifestyle?

3. Do you analyze your food or activity journal to learn the reasons for your successes and challenges?

4. Do you eat three meals each day every three to four hours? If not, what gets in your way?

5. Do your meals include a protein, vegetables, and a small amount of starchy carbs, or does your plate look like shades of beige?

6. Do you eat planned snacks, or do you find yourself grazing between meals?

7. Can you sense when you've had enough to eat *before* you overdo it?

8. Are you able to tell the difference between cravings and <u>actual</u> hunger?

9. Does boredom, frustration or other uncomfortable feelings drive you to eat?

10. Do you have a list of enjoyable activities that you do between meals instead of filling the time snacking and eating mindlessly?

11. Do you make regular changes in your diet and lifestyle based on information you've gathered about weight, eating habits and physical activity, or do you change your habits because you've seen something work for someone else?

Weight-Loss Goals

Our second tool is a familiar one: weight-loss goals. And I mean more than just the scale.

I joke that I could probably produce the next hit reality show if I placed a hidden camera on our clinic scales. If only these machines could talk. I see beautiful, confident women hold their breath and tremble when they step toward this device. Grown men look away as if something scary is going to jump out. I've seen tears of sorrow. I've seen explosions of joy. I've seen avoidance. I've seen people weigh in two or three times a day.

So now, we'll start using the scale for what it is – a measuring tool. It will be one of many tools that we'll use to collect data to help us make decisions. This is a huge shift for many people. But freedom starts when our emotions are controlled by us – not a scale.

Begin by setting the goal(s) for your weight loss. I know, you're probably thinking, "Isn't weight loss the goal?" Sure, losing weight is important, and so is keeping it off. But what, other than a lighter body, will the weight loss bring you? What if your goal is to breathe better? To move more with less pain? To gain confidence? Or maybe to help you get promoted or enjoy your children? There are lots of reasons to lose weight. What's important are YOUR reasons. This exercise will help you identify your PERSONAL goals for weight loss.

Obesity affects people in different ways. Not all people who are obese have medical problems – but many do. Are you healthy except for your excess weight? Are you struggling with health problems? List the health goals that you most want to achieve. Talk with your medical team about these challenges to be sure you set realistic goals and expectations as you lose weight.

Excess weight can make simple daily activities difficult. How does your weight affect your daily life? What activities are you hoping to do as you lose weight?

Often people say they want to lose weight so they can be HAPPIER. What does happy mean for you? What HAVEN'T you been able to achieve in your life because of your excess weight? What would be your top three personal goals that you want to achieve as a result of your weight loss?

There's no ideal weight or chart that can say what success should be for you. Only you and your medical team can decide that. Dr. Arya Sharma, a prominent obesity researcher at the University of Alberta, proposes, "Your best weight is going to be the one you can maintain while having a healthy, enjoyable life."

A Word About Body Mass Index (BMI)

We've all heard the term "BMI," and now that you're on the My Hungry Head journey, you may be wondering how important it is to you.

The answer: Probably not very important.

BMI, which stands for Body Mass Index, is widely used as a screening tool to indicate whether a person is underweight, overweight, obese, or a healthy weight for their height. But it may not be as helpful as we think, mostly because it fails to account for natural variations in individuals. And it can lend itself to the "one size fits all" approach that My Hungry Head is designed to avoid.

During an interview on the NPR show *Your Health*, mathematician Keith Devlin explained that the BMI was introduced in the early 19th century by a Belgian named Lambert Adolphe Jacques Quetelet. He was a mathematician, not a physician. He produced the formula to give a quick and easy way to measure the degree of obesity of the general population to assist the government in allocating resources. In other words, Devlin says, "it is a 200-year-old hack."

BMI makes no allowance for the relative proportions of bone, muscle, and fat in the body. But bone is denser than muscle and twice as dense as fat, so a person with strong bones, good muscle tone and low fat will have a high BMI. So many athletes, for example, may find themselves classified as overweight or even obese.

Because most people today lead fairly sedentary lives and are not particularly active, the formula tacitly assumes low muscle mass and high relative fat content. It applies moderately well when applied to such people because it was formulated by focusing on them. But it gives exactly the wrong answer for a large and significant section of the population, namely the lean, fit, and healthy. Quetelet is also the person who came up with the idea of "the average man." That's a useful concept, but if you try to apply it to any one person, you come up with the absurdity of a person with 2.4 children. Averages measure entire populations and often don't apply to individuals. BMI is simply a ratio of weight in relation to height. It is not a direct measurement of body fat. And this is important: This ratio provides no information about distribution of body fat.

In contrast, comparing hip and waist circumference provides information about where body fat is stored. Waist-to-hip ratio is *simply a measurement of waist size compared to hip size. It is an important measurement because it is a good indicator of visceral fat, which resides in the abdominal area and is more closely linked to chronic diseases such as coronary heart disease, hypertension and diabetes.*

So how do you know what your body is made up of? There are lots of ways to measure body composition. Some are expensive and hard-to-find such as DEXA Scans, Plethysmography (BodPod) and hydro-static or underwater weighing. Others are quick and easy such as bio-impedance. Impedance scales use faint electrical impulses that run through your body. The theory is that fat will block or that run through your body. Muscle will allow it to travel quickly.

Source: Keith Devlin, Your Health radio show, NPR. July 4, 2009

Create your own personal Success Monitor – the set of goals you want to achieve. Additionally, talk with your medical team and those close to you about what you hope to achieve. At some point, the number on the scale will stop moving and you will have to define success in other ways. Use your success monitor as a reminder of what you've really achieved!

Success doesn't just happen. Before you get started, let's think about making room for success.

Let's start with why now? What is your motivation to get your Hungry Head under control?

Unfortunately, motivation won't be enough. Ask any Olympic athlete or successful musician. Look behind any achievement, and you'll find lots of practice, focus and a heavy dose of perseverance.

Set yourself up for success now.

Identify the person you will turn to for support. Having people around us who believe in us and want us to succeed is crucial. Make a list of those people in your life. Some may already be there, and some you might have to find.

These people may be family members, friends, colleagues, local weight-loss groups or online forums such as My Hungry Head's.

My Body Composition

Body fat % _____
Fat free mass _____
Waist Circumference _____
Hip Circumference _____
Hip to Waist Ratio = Waist/Hip _____

My Health Goals

☐ Lower Blood Pressure   ☐ Improve Sleep Apnea
☐ Increase HDL Good Cholesterol   ☐ Decrease Joint Pain
☐ Decrease LDL Bad Cholesterol   ☐ Improve Breathing
☐ Lower Blood Sugar   ☐ Decrease Anxiety
                                      ☐ Decrease Depression

My Personal Goals

What do I want to do with my improved health?

1. _____
   _____
   _____

2. _____
   _____
   _____

3. _____
   _____
   _____

Talk to your healthcare provider about you body composition goals and health goals. Be sure these goals are realistic and achievable safely.

Lastly, create space and time in your schedule that you will devote to practicing My Hungry Head mastery steps. Where will you take your courses? How will you make time to practice your steps to success? Some of these will happen naturally during your day, and some you will need to schedule in.

As we unpack the tools, set aside time in your schedule to read, understand, and contemplate how the My Hungry Head Mindset & Mastery Steps make sense for you.

Remember, you may have to give something up to make time for your My Hungry Head program. This is part of getting honest. Are you willing to commit your time and energy in order to have lasting success?

The next chapters will cover the six critical skills needed to stabilize your weight.

- Objectively observing facts and data.
- Analyzing your hunger cycle.
- Identifying real hunger vs. emotional hunger.
- Retraining your brain with a productive message.
- Generating new ideas to improve life between meals.
- Taking a big-picture approach to identifying the right problem and solutions.

Abby's Story

Abby, 29, was a stay-at-home mom. She married Brad, her high school sweetheart. While Brad works full-time, Abby cares for their 7-year-old daughter and 5-year-old son.

Battling post-partum depression, Abby had gained weight after the birth of her first child.

A worrier by nature, she tended to need reassurance when meeting life's challenges, and losing weight would be no exception. She came from a broken home, and this made it all the more important for her to feel that she was a good wife and mother.

Abby often made home-cooked dinners, but struggled throughout the day while her kids were in school. She cycled through salty-crunchy snacks and cookies and cupcakes, grabbing bits and pieces as she moved through her day.

"I just don't have enough time to make breakfast and lunch for myself," she said in her first My Hungry Head class. "By the time I get my kids off to school, I have to rush to get my house in order before the son gets off the kindergarten bus."

She had no significant support other than her husband and a close friend.

Like most of my patients, Abby came to me ready to lose weight. She said she wanted to change. Specifically, I learned, this meant that she wanted to change her size. She was tired of feeling heavy and lethargic, which she attributed to her weight. She wanted to feel athletic and energetic again.

What wasn't clear was what Abby was willing to do to achieve these goals.

She wanted to prove to her husband that she could do this. She could lose the weight once and for all and show him she could be a fun-loving wife and mom. She was down on herself, and her self-imposed pressure to get the weight off was creating unnecessary anxiety.

I needed to help her slow down, identify her strengths, and build up the areas in which she struggled.

"I'll be honest. When I first found out I had to get my emotions and my house in order to get this weight off, I got a bit discouraged," she said. "Taking the My Hungry Head program seemed like another impossible task for me to complete, another obstacle. I just wanted to know what I should eat to lose weight. But I knew others who went to the program. I wanted their calmness, too. So I did the steps."

In the "Making Room for Success" step, Abby accepted that she couldn't do this on her own. She couldn't diet by day for six weeks, then surprise her husband with a 20-pound weight loss. If she was going to lose this weight and keep it off, she needed him on this journey.

This involved Abby identifying what she needed from Brad. This included:

- *Watching the kids one night a week to attend class.*
- *Accompanying her on family walks after dinner.*
- *Getting him and the kids to accept the need to decrease the amount of processed food and sugary snacks in the house.*

She also needed to make time for herself to quiet down and settle into her day, with a task list, rather than rushing and reacting. In about eight weeks, by meeting these small-step goals, she lost 28 pounds.

"Some days are tough," she said, "but most are really easy now and very free-flowing. After losing 28 pounds, I feel like there's nothing I can't do. I feel as if my *hungry head* is now my *happy head*. Life couldn't be better. My husband and I are so thankful."

CHAPTER 3

The Objective
Observer

*The greatest value of a picture is
when it forces us to notice
what we never expected to see.*

– JOHN TUKEY

n this chapter, we'll examine two key tools for controlling weight: a personal food journal and a scale. Most important, we'll learn how to benefit from them rather than let them drive us crazy.

Let's start with journaling.

Some people love it and some hate it. For a long time, I didn't understand it, at least not as a weight-control aid. I wondered, "What's the point of writing down what I ate AFTER eating it? What good is a list of stuff that is already in my body? I was already feeling bad enough, now I have to relive it?!"

In my desperation for a tool to control my weight, I did dutifully record all my meals, snacks and indulgences. Again and again. Counting calories or fat or carbs – whatever diet I was on at the time – never doing any more with the information than that. Although I was writing down what I ate, I was not really OBSERVING.

Learning to observe ourselves is one of the most important skills you will learn in My Hungry Head. Becoming an objective observer of your own behavior is the first step to becoming the master of it. Neutral observation will help you get to know the internal and external factors pulling and pushing you toward eating, the patterns, feelings and emotions involved in our eating. And you'll learn what actually works for you.

So many of us **trapped in the diet prison** have spent years looking outside of ourselves for advice on how to get skinny or healthy. You don't have to look far to find some magazine or TV doctor touting the best way for *you* to manage *your* weight. We've ALL spent years trying to follow generic weight-loss plans for our unique bodies. And then we feel bad about ourselves because they don't work for us. Now it's time to observe what works for you and what doesn't.

So, how do you feel about using a food journal? Do you already use one? Once a week? Once a month? Or maybe never?

If you answered every day, then great! It sounds like you don't mind journaling at all! You're probably recording what you eat and how much you eat. You're off to a great start.

If you answered that you are journaling once a week or less, we will invite you to make it a regular practice as we begin to bring awareness to eating habits and food choices.

If you answered never, then we invite you to step into the world of journaling, if only in this beginning part of your journey. Who knows, you may enjoy getting honest with yourself and your journal.

You don't have to journal every day forever, if it's not your thing, but some strategic journaling at the onset will take you a long way.

Start small if you need to. Journaling a couple of days during the week and one day on the weekend should be enough to get you started.

Deciding what you want to use to journal and track yourself is important. Are you someone who likes to write on paper, or do you prefer a digital device such as your smartphone or tablet? If you like to handwrite, get a journal that is small enough to carry around with you so that you can have it with you at all times. If you want to use a digital device, you can find tools to track your eating and activity on your smartphone or online. Make it as easy for yourself as possible.

Track what and how much you eat, when and where you eat, how long it takes, and what you feel like. What are your cravings like? Your energy? Your hunger? What is your mood like?

Some people find that they had no idea how much they were eating or that they were really anxious before every meal in which they overate or that when they ate late at night they felt more out of control.

Let's break it down: *What should you write in your journal?*

For starters, you'll want to collect information about what and how much you eat.

Do your best to estimate the actual portion size. You may need to get a small food scale to be sure your portion sizes are on target. It's not uncommon for many of us to have to recalibrate our perception of portion sizes. Thanks to value meals, supersizing and typical restaurant portions, we've all suffered from distorted portions.

Food packages may tell you how much a portion is, but what you *think* is a half-cup and what is *actually* a half-cup may be totally different. It's funny how a half-cup of cooked spinach can look different from a half-cup of mocha ice cream! If you're addicted to ice cream, I'll bet that half-cup of creamy mocha is bigger ... right? And of course fresh fruits and vegetables have no indicator.

So get real and honest about the amount of food you are eating. We'll be most interested in tracking macronutrients such as protein, carbohydrates and fiber. For now, we will not be as concerned with the calorie count as with WHAT makes up those calories. Let's face it, 1,200 calories of lean protein and veggies will affect your body radically differently than 1,200 calories of gummy bears and martinis.

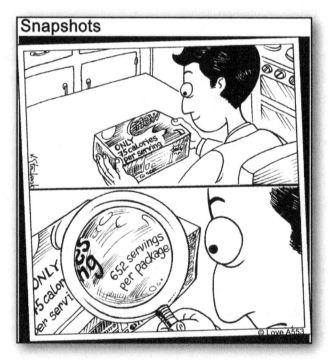

Now for the real game-changing data.

Identifying **when** you eat and the **context** around your meals and snacks will be just as important as what you eat. There are many, many reasons that we overeat. Some may be physical urges, emotional triggers or social pressures. Much of why we eat has very little to do with willpower.

You'll learn in the next chapter, *The Hunger Cycle*, that your body has a unique rhythm of hunger and satiety, or sense of fullness. The data you collect now will help you figure out how to manage your unique rhythm of hunger.

For each meal or snack, start tracking this information:

- *What time was your meal?*
- *Where did you eat? At the table, TV, car, desk?*
- *Who were you eating with?*
- *How fast or slowly did you eat?*
- *Can you recall the taste or texture of your food?*
- *What was your mood like?*
- *Why were you eating?*
- *What were your hunger, energy and cravings like before you ate?*

Notice if you automatically start judging yourself about any of these facts you are tracking. If you are, make note of that, too.

There's no judgment to be passed on the data you collect. There's no perfect plan to follow. For now, you are just being a detective, gathering neutral information to help you make better decisions.

Imagine you are helping a good friend gather information to make an important decision. You don't want to influence her or hurt her in any way. Of course you wouldn't say hurtful things to your friends. You wouldn't tell a stranger he or she is fat, would you? Why do that to yourself? You're just collecting the facts. And the facts might include something like "When I ate late at night, I felt guilty." Even though it is about a feeling, your experience is a fact.

Remember, this is a practice. If you find yourself writing what you had for lunch and then admonishing yourself for eating too much or what you consider to be the "wrong" things, that is a judgment. If you congratulate yourself on eating less than you wanted or eating the "right" foods, that is a judgment, too!

It isn't easy, but journaling with a neutral attitude, no matter what you are documenting, is a valuable skill. Keep at it and bear in mind that no one ever lost an ounce by beating themselves up. If you feel you must add some emotion, try adding curiosity.

Non-Judgmental Weigh-Ins

The scale gives us information to help us guide our behavior. That's it! The manufacturers of your scale did not design it to make you feel good or bad. They don't know you! Only you make yourself feel bad. Negative messages serve absolutely no purpose. They create unnecessary anxiety and take our focus away from achieving our real goals.

Our basic view on using a scale is this: Stepping on a scale is a way to know where our weight is. It's OK to weigh yourself every day as long as the number on the scale doesn't control your mood. Ideally, weigh yourself at the same time of the day. For our purposes, we will only write down our weight once a week. Pick any day that works for you, but keep it the same each week. Some people like weighing first thing in the morning "because I'll weigh less." It doesn't really matter whether you weigh in the morning or evening – just use the same scale around the same time of day. You are looking for trends week to week – not daily or hourly.

If your mood is affected by discovering daily shifts in water weight, de-crease your stress by only weighing yourself once each week on the day you will be writing it down. It is normal for your weight to fluctuate a few pounds due to water shifts. Remember, you are looking for fat loss, not small shifts in water weight.

If you haven't stepped on a scale for months, don't worry about it. Just start weighing yourself once each week. I've worked with many patients who want avoid the scale because they "just don't want to know." I've learned most patients know where they stand with their weight. I know, it's hard to step on that scale. The number is a tally of our behavior, some of which we don't want to be reminded about. But think about it ... you already know what you've done.

It's easy for your weight to slowly slip out of hand if you're not paying attention. Weighing can serve as a valuable tool to help us manage our weight – if we don't let it affect our mood. Research suggests people who weigh themselves regularly are more successful at managing their weight than those who don't.

Again, as with journaling, observe and write down not just your weight, but how weighing yourself affects you. Find the best frequency for you – but no more than once a day and no less than once a week.

Kristen's Story

Kristen came to me because she was worried that she was putting on weight. She was a thin, attractive brunette. She never struggled with her weight and was always thin up until the arrival of her first child 15 years earlier. Once children arrived, an active social life gave way to the day-to-day responsibilities of managing her time as a working mother.

Her goal for coming to me? To lose weight. "I want to be 135 pounds, and I don't know why I'm not losing weight. I'm trying so hard. I eat really well, but I can't figure out why I always feel so terrible AND I can't move the scale. I weigh myself every day. It's driving me crazy. I never eat more calories than I need; most of the time I have calories left over. What's wrong with me? I need help." Kristen obsessed about reaching this goal. It was her first thought in the morning and it continued haunting her throughout the day.

Kristen accounted for everything she put in her mouth. Every morsel of food was recorded in her calorie tracker app, which made our job easier. The results were just as Kristen had said: According to her food tracker, she rarely ate any more than the calories her body needed.

It was time for Kristen to "up" her observation skills. In order to help her, we needed to figure out not just what she was eating, but when, where and why.

A few more days of journaling showed us that when Kristen ate meals, they were generally pretty healthy. She could make good food choices, but didn't always eat at regular times. She often skipped lunch due to her stressful schedule at work. By the time she came home, she was wound tight and needed to relax.

While cooking dinner, she would have a couple of martinis, though she was always careful to use only sugar-free mixers.

Between meals, she ate candy – throughout the day – but only "fat-free candy – NEVER chocolate. I know the difference." She never traveled without the candy. There it was, a large bag of gummy bears peeking out of her purse.

"I'm tired all the time. They're the only thing that keep me awake during the day. I eat them all the time, but I account for them. I recorded every one of them in my journal. They're fat-free, they shouldn't make a difference."

Kristen was honest. She never lied to me, or to herself. She just couldn't grasp the causes behind her eating or why she felt so tired and unwell.

Kristen had spent the last 15 years dieting. She could count calories better than anyone else I knew. She was an obsessive food-tracker. But although she could count well, she was missing vital clues as to how her body and mind could feel better.

Our first step was to help Kristen wrestle free from the diets holding her hostage. Her mind was cluttered with a tangled web of diet advice – some good, some bad – that she had collected over the years. Rather than making the calorie math add up, we needed to learn what makes Kristen feel alive and satisfied throughout the day. She needed to use food journals in a new way.

Kristen did well adjusting to our new approach to journaling. Suddenly she was paying attention to the unnecessary distractions at work that kept her from lunch. It was becoming clear how little she ate at dinner because she felt tired and woozy after the two or three martinis she needed to calm herself down after work. After a couple of weeks, much to her surprise, Kristen was entering insightful information in her journal without flogging herself. She even stopped balancing her caloric checkbook!

Now it was time to address her obsessive visits to the scale. Kristen had plenty of stress going on in her life. Her obsession with the scale was only making things worse. She was weighing herself daily, sometimes several times a day.

Every minor shift in her weight – one, two, or three pounds – drove her crazy. For Kristen, it was 135 pounds or bust.

Before I could even start helping Kristen, I needed to understand whether 135 pounds was a healthy, achievable goal for her. Next, I had to understand what was REALLY important to her. She was in good health; she had no signs of high blood pressure, high cholesterol, diabetes or any other medical issues. Did she want to *feel* smaller? More fit? More active? Or did she just want to be 135 pounds?

I remember how confused she looked when I asked these questions. "What the hell is the difference? Why does it matter?" she asked.

I started with a body composition analysis using an impedance scale to identify what made up Kristen's current weight. We measured her total body fat, fat-free body mass, and total body water. We would do this weekly to track changes over the next several weeks and identify whether water or fat accounted for any weight changes.

43

We learned from the body composition analysis that Kristen's total body fat was high for a slightly active female her age. This meant she had less lean, energy-burning (or calorie-burning) muscle mass. Kristen was what we consider "skinny fat" – someone who is not overweight and has a "skinny" look, but still has a high percentage of body fat and low muscle mass.

Our data collection process would help us figure out what Kristen needed to change in her diet and what lifestyle adjustments she could make to increase her lean muscle mass. Kristen eventually accepted that she needed to measure success differently. It wasn't easy, but she slowly began to set her sights on other goals.

Her personal Success Monitor changed from "wanting to weigh 135 pounds" to being able to have more energy to live her life, to let go of all the mental energy keeping her imprisoned in her calorie-counting and to figure out how to have more time in her day to take care of her nutritional needs.

Once Kristen was able to stabilize her eating patterns, she set her sights on fixing the real problem – her work situation. Rather than obsessing about weighing 135 pounds, Kristen spent her energy implementing a well-crafted job search.

The Objective Observer Mindset

Sometimes one statement can change your mind forever. This happened to me when I read James McBride's memoir, *The Color of Water: A Black Man's Tribute to His White Mother.*

As a young boy, McBride was searching for his place, where he fit in the world, when he asked his mother whether God was black or white. She said God was neither black nor white, but rather a spirit. "What color is God's spirit?" McBride persisted. In a time of racial tension and prejudice, his mother responded with a powerful, yet simple statement: "God is the color of water. Water doesn't have a color." Nowhere in her statement could you hear any judgment about being black or white, rich or poor, good or bad.

Water has no color. Think of the color of water when you are collecting facts and information about your weight and eating behavior. Observe yourself without making judgments – good or bad. Simply record what you weigh, what you eat, and the context around your eating behavior. Just the facts.

Stop the old diet commentary running in your head when you step on the scale or record in your food journal. You're now a neutral observer collecting facts and information to improve yourself. There will be plenty of time to deal with emotions. For now, each time that critical voice pops up, stop!

Tell yourself:
"I am an investigator searching for clues.
I have a goal.
I need information to help me decide how
I will achieve my goal.
The information I collect is not a statement
of who I am as a person."

Mastery Steps

- Begin weighing and recording your weight weekly. Do NOT step on the scale more than once a week if doing so negatively affects your mood.
- Get a body composition analysis if you can. Purchase a home impedance scale if you'd like to monitor your body fat.
- Note week-to-week weight changes, NOT daily changes.
- Using the Objective Observer Tool Sheet, create a food journal at least three days per week and one day on the weekend.
- Just collect the facts. NO judgment.
- Go gently! The goal of this Mindset and Mastery Step is to help your brain break free from the emotional roller coaster of high hopes and broken weight-loss dreams. It will take practice.

CHAPTER 4

Your Hunger Cycle

I try to feed my hunger rather than my appetite.

– GINGER ROGERS

n this chapter, we will learn how to analyze the information we have gathered this week on weight, diet and activity. This is not to make you feel bad or, for that matter, overly confident. It's to figure out where you can make improvements.

First, let's learn about the hunger cycle in the body and how you can use this information to manage your own Hungry Head.

The Body's Adaptive System

Let's start with looking at what our bodies are designed to do. Some theories say that we're actually designed to binge on food when it is available. Thousands of years ago, when most people still lived in hunter/gatherer communities, there were times when food was scarce. Feast or famine was real.

We had to eat as much food as we could find and store the extra calories, or energy, as fat for times of scarcity. Those whose bodies were good at storing fat would have quite the evolutionary advantage during times of famine.

Fast-forward a few thousand years, and in many parts of the world, food is everywhere. Many of us barely have to move to get food. And yet, our bodies have not evolved to reflect this. Other factors that have changed are the kinds of food that are available and the additives and preservatives in them that our bodies were never made to process.

What's more, many processed foods and convenience foods on supermarket shelves are designed to make us crave more of them.

Some of these foods are obviously "junk," but others are sold as being healthy. And if these foods are designed to make us want more, how can we keep from bingeing? Especially if our bodies are designed to eat food when it is available and to become addicted to certain kinds of substances that are now in so many processed foods.

The key is learning to sort out the messages that were programmed into us thousands of years ago to keep us healthy from those that bombard us from supermarket shelves, fast food restaurants, TV commercials and other realities of the 21st century.

When we're eating food that is addictive and makes us feel out of control, our bodies will send us the message that we need more of it. However, this is not the hunger response calling out, but the chemical dependency on this type of food. Our bodies may be craving real nutrition, but that signal is overridden by the addictive nature of processed foods high in salt, sugar and unhealthy fats.

Anyone who has been to a Walt Disney theme park knows how difficult it is to eat right when you're there – let alone get our kids to eat right.

Marketing magic starts the second you cross into the "Happiest Place on Earth." We learned this on a family vacation to Disney World. By the time we drove to the park from our hotel and rode Pluto's shuttle to the front gate, any satiety from breakfast was wearing off. The second we hit Main Street, we began salivating at the sights and smells of old-fashioned cookies. This was no accident.

And have you ever noticed how TV commercials for food usually start a couple of hours after the normal dinner hour?

This world filled with convenience food has created a mindset that we are entitled to have food available quickly. We feel put out if we actually have to spend time prepping and cooking food. We feel that we are entitled to eat candy and cake and that not eating these foods is a kind of deprivation.

Perhaps this is partly due to the dependence created by sugar, salt, fat and other chemicals in processed food, but it is also due to a mindset that we are entitled to have these foods. When did a "treat" become a necessity? I want to invite you to entertain the possibility that perhaps these convenient treats and ultra-processed foods might be bringing you little or no nutrition at all. In other words, they may not be real food. Get your mind around that.

The Decision to Eat

With food everywhere and available at all times of the day, we've got to get really good at understanding WHEN to eat and when NOT to eat. How do we get our real hunger cycle back in working order?

Obviously, food gives us the energy and the fuel our body uses to grow, move and thrive. Our bodies have a very sophisticated system to help us regulate this energy. They communicate to us via sensation. By learning to listen to our bodies, we can tune in to the messages that come from real need and not from the craving mind.

Let's look at how this body alert system affects your urge to eat.

First, your body uses hunger PANGS to start the hunger cycle. This is caused by hydrochloric acid churning in your stomach. You may notice a burning sensation, a hollow feeling or growling.

If you don't listen to your hunger pangs or miss their message, your body will send another round of communication. This time, it heightens your senses. Now food may start smelling better or maybe it starts looking more attractive.

If you don't respond to your hunger pangs or heightened senses, your body will use another layer of communication – hormones – to get you to eat. Think of hormones as your body's messengers. One of those hormones, ghrelin, is like a cute little monster just looking for attention. Here to help, its job is to get you to eat. Ignore it and it will just scream louder and louder. Ever feel like you could eat your arm off after skipping meals? Well, that's ghrelin hard at work. Known as "the hunger hormone," it gradually increases before meals. It's found mostly in the stomach and scurries up to your brain by way of the vagus nerve to remind you to eat.

Once you've had a meal, your stomach will do some extra stretching to digest your food. These muscular contractions and movements helps push your food along, but they also stimulate more communication between your stomach and your brain, telling your brain that you have had a meal and have satisfied your hunger.

Cholecystokinin (CCK) may be one of those hormones stimulated by stomach stretching. CCK sends a message that says "I've had enough for now." Its job is to get you to stop eating. The trouble is that CCK can be a fleeting messenger.

If you're eating too fast or not paying attention, you may miss the "I've had enough" cue. But don't worry, the body's communication system is pretty sophisticated. If you miss a cue, more messengers are produced as your food moves through your intestines. Peptide YY and GLP-1 are more hormonal messengers available to get you to stop eating. CCK, PYY, GLP-1 ... there's no need to worry about who's who at the hormone and peptide party. All you need to know is that these guys are working hard in your intestine, just to let you know when to stop eating. Ignore them and you'll likely take in more energy – or food – than your body needs.

Leptin is another hormone that has emerged as a big player in the feeling-full game. Leptin moves a little slower than your other gut hormones, but it also does a little extra work. In addition to quieting appetite signals, leptin is also involved in fat storage. It plays a big role in quieting the appetite signal in your brain. Leptin likes good sleep – not enough and you may find yourself short on this hormone and therefore having less of that satisfied feeling after you eat.

Planned Eating

Now that you know how the hunger cycle works, your job is to start working with your hunger cues, not against them. It's time to say good-bye to meal-skipping and hello to regular meals and planned snacks. Planned eating is a key element in controlling your hungry head.

Work on eating three meals each day, about three to four hours apart, with a couple of planned snacks in between. Even if you do not hear your body's hunger signals now because of years of overriding them, you will regain the ability to hear your hunger cycle alert system by eating in a regular, consistent way.

We want to stress the word "planned" here. This may mean preparing your own food and bringing it to work or planning strategically about when, where or how you go out to eat. It's easy to eat more than we need when our hunger is out of control from meal-skipping or racing through our day without a plan.

People who skip breakfast, and meals in general, leave space for hunger hormones to be so loud and out of sync that when we eat, we may feel like we can't stop.

What to Eat

My mom always put together a colorful plate, using plenty of fruits and vegetables. It looked pretty, but that wasn't the point: It was a sign that the meal was balanced.

We should all strive for this, even if the food isn't literally on one plate. Obviously, salad and fruit are often served as side dishes. And you can even have "Mom's plate" on a sandwich!

So what should go on your "plate"? Try to have a plate that is half veggies. One quarter of your plate should be a good source of protein, such as meat, poultry or fish, and the remaining quarter of your plate should have a small amount of starchy carbs.

You won't need a lot of protein – about four to five ounces per meal should be enough. If you've had weight-loss surgery, you may only be able to tolerate smaller portions, perhaps only two ounces at a time.

Protein moves more slowly through your digestive system, helping your body release those hormones and peptides that tell your brain to decrease your appetite and cravings. Solid protein requires more contractions by the intestines to process, which in turn may release more CCK, the first "you've had enough" message. Be sure to eat your protein first, especially if you've had weight-loss surgery, because this is the only nutrient you cannot replace with a vitamin.

You can eat plenty of vegetables, at least half a plate. Fruits are fine to eat with your meals, but just don't overdo it. Less-sweet fruits such as apples, pears and berries are a great start. Because fruits contain natural sugar, you may want to reserve them for a snack or dessert. Your goal with vegetables and fruits is to create a plate that is colorful, packed with a variety of nutrients. If your plate is mostly brown and beige, you're on the wrong track!

Starchy carbohydrates, such as potatoes, pasta, rice and bread are tricky. You'll need to watch the amount of these carbs you take in. *Too much* will slow your weight loss, or perhaps cause weight gain. *Too little* and you may feel tired and sluggish. Keep in mind that you'll be getting plenty of carbohydrates from vegetables and fruits, so you won't need a whole lot of starchy carbs.

A small amount (e.g., a tablespoon) of healthy fat such as olive oil, coconut oil, avocado, olives and nuts may actually aid in lowering "bad" cholesterol. But remember, just because they are "good" fats doesn't mean you can have a lot. Treat these tasty accoutrements as a finishing touch – do not overdo it.

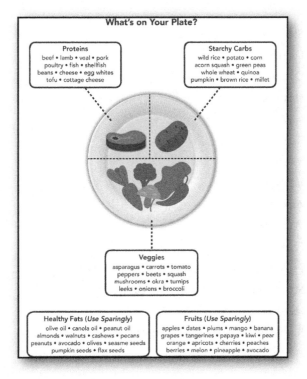

What's on Your Plate?

Proteins
beef • lamb • veal • pork
poultry • fish • shellfish
beans • cheese • egg whites
tofu • cottage cheese

Starchy Carbs
wild rice • potato • corn
acorn squash • green peas
whole wheat • quinoa
pumpkin • brown rice • millet

Veggies
asparagus • carrots • tomato
peppers • beets • squash
mushrooms • okra • turnips
leeks • onions • broccoli

Healthy Fats (*Use Sparingly*)
olive oil • canola oil • peanut oil
almonds • walnuts • cashews • pecans
peanuts • avocado • olives • seasme seeds
pumpkin seeds • flax seeds

Fruits (*Use Sparingly*)
apples • dates • plums • mango • banana
grapes • tangerines • papaya • kiwi • pear
orange • apricots • cherries • peaches
berries • melon • pineapple • avocado

What **NOT** to Eat

Unlike most diets, we don't specify what you should eat. Even if we did tell you what to eat, after a while, you would just eat what you want anyway. That's why prescribed diets don't work. The My Hungry Head program wants you to choose what you'd like to eat based on your taste and preferences.

Keeping true to the allotted portions for protein, starchy carbs and vegetables will take you a long way to ensuring that you get the right amount of nutrients for your body. The only foods you should avoid are those that make you feel sick OR out of control.

Feeling sick can mean different things for different people. Here are some typical signs that indicate you may want to avoid a certain food:

- Bloating
- Diarrhea
- Dizziness
- Heart palpitations
- Nausea
- Rapid heart rate
- Sweating
- Vomiting
- Anxiety
- Weakness
- Fatigue
- Problems concentrating or feeling confused
- Strong feelings of hunger after eating
- Headaches or migraines
- Rashes, eczema or other allergies

You may have certain "trigger" foods that you may want to eliminate until you have stabilized your eating patterns. Which foods should you eliminate? To create the best chance of success for yourself, eliminate those foods that cause you to lose control over your portions.

Like feeling "sick," losing control is also dependent on each person. I could have 10 gallons of ice cream in my freezer and never give it a second thought. But give me a bag of Lay's potato chips, and I can prove in no time why their tagline, "Betcha can't eat just one," is a fact.

Here are some clues that you may be losing control:

- Eating large amounts of food, even when not physically hungry.
- Unable to stop eating when you want to.
- Unable to control how much you are eating.
- Eating unplanned meal or snacks.
- Eating rapidly during binge episodes.
- Eating until you're uncomfortably full.
- Frequently eating alone or in secret.
- Hiding food.
- Embarrassment at the quantity of food being eaten.
- Feeling depressed, disgusted, ashamed, or guilty about your eating.
- Frequently dieting, possibly without weight loss.
- Vomiting after eating.
- Excessive exercise.
- Gaining more than 10 pounds in a short period of time.

What About Snacking?

There's nothing wrong with having a snack. Yes, I repeat, there's nothing wrong with snacking! The only problem with snacking comes when we can't stop. Or when we replace meals with snacks. If you are eating a balanced meal every three to four hours, you may need or want a small snack in between. One or two planned snacks during the day can be useful – and enjoyable.

The guidelines for snacking are the same as for meals. Eat whatever you'd like as long as it doesn't make you sick AND you have control. Make your life easier. Identify the foods that trigger your binge behavior and remove them from your house. It's going to be infinitely more difficult to manage your hungry head with these temptations all around you. Think about it ... alcoholics don't get sober in bars.

Snacks are more satisfying when they include a protein. Now I'm not talking about a burger and fries. The snacks I'm talking about are just that, "snack" portions that will fit into a half-cup size ramekin bowl.

But let's be real. Who's going to feel satisfied by 12 potato chips in a half-cup bowl? Not many of us. Most refined carbohydrates like chips, pretzels, crackers, cakes and cookies melt easily and take little effort for our bodies to digest. These treats cause very little contractions in your digestive system – which means less "I've had enough" chemicals release to the brain.

For the best bang-for-your-buck snacking, combine your crunchy carbs with a protein or healthy fat. Get creative with taste-boosters such as fresh herbs, spices and condiments.

Here are some ideas:

Upgrade Your Snacks

Carb n' Crunch	+	Protein & Healthy Fat	+	Taste Upgrade
pretzel log	+	deli turkey/roast beef	+	dijon mustard
pear	+	crushed almonds	+	gorgonzola cheese
melba toast	+	ricotta cheese	+	honey drizzle
apple	+	peanut butter	+	toasted coconut
flatbread cracker	+	avocado	+	fresh salsa
celery	+	low-fat cream cheese	+	kalamata olives
banana	+	crushed peanuts	+	cocoa powder
toasted mini-bagel	+	low-fat cream cheese	+	cherries
popcorn	+	parmesan cheese	+	cayenne pepper
wasa cracker	+	smoked salmon	+	tomatoes & capers
rice cracker	+	edamame spread	+	ginger & soy
strawberries	+	brie cheese	+	balsamic & basil
watermelon	+	feta cheese	+	balsamic & mint
crisp flatbread	+	feta cheese	+	marinated olives
grapes	+	chicken salad	+	curry powder
tomato	+	tuna salad	+	capers

Size Matters

When we were talking about what to eat, we had you visualize a plate. When considering the real plates in your kitchen, here's another strategy to help you with portion control: Get rid of those 10.5-inch monsters, let alone the tire-sized ones you sometimes find in restaurants. They only encourage you to eat more. Start with a salad plate or small dinner plate for your meals.

Our Growing Dinner Plate

In an article called Dishing Yourself into a Smaller Size, Dr. Pamela Peeke noted that a typical dinner plate size in the 1960s was nine inches and that it had increased gradually over the years to today's 12 inches. So it's grown from about 64 square inches to about 113 square inches – nearly doubling the amount of calories a plate can hold!

In my own household, going back down to nine-inch plates caused a few waves at the family table. My husband and sons mocked right-sized portions, calling dinner "the new snack." Eventually their full stomachs convinced them we were all eating "enough."

But the biggest backlash was about the all-purpose soup-to-cereal ice cream bowls.

Although I was relieved that we didn't eat ice cream out of the container, the bowls could hold five scoops of Rocky Road with room to spare. That's a whopping 750 calories, close to half of what my body needs for an entire day. Not to mention the 40 grams of saturated fat and more carbohydrates than I needed.

With some grumbling, my family adjusted to new ramekin-size cups. And, no, filling them with M&Ms was unacceptable.

When I show my patients a comparison of plate sizes, they are always shocked at the calorie difference that one inch in diameter can make.

Environment Matters

Eat in a calm environment when possible, and take your time. This may feel very new for you, so many of us are used to eating fast and in stressful environments. Journaling should be making it easier for you to recognize this. Making the effort to bring calm and relaxation to your eating will not only help you hear the messages of satiety from your body, but it will help you digest your food better by cutting down on the stress hormone, cortisol, that can contribute to increased appetite.

This may mean turning off the television, which keeps you from concentrating on what you're eating even if the program you're watching isn't particularly stressful. Also avoid eating in your car or on the run, and you might even consider avoiding eating with certain people in your life.

If you cannot eat every meal in a calm environment, practice taking some full deep breaths before you begin your meal. Notice the colors, the textures, the flavors. Paying attention to what you are eating goes a long way toward calming your mind.

When considering the "I don't have time to eat" situations that some of us find ourselves in, let's face it: Most are self-created. Most things in life can wait 30 minutes without a catastrophe happening. It's not like everyone with eating difficulties is a first responder called to an emergency – or a surgeon who can't leave a patient on the operating table. Sure, what we do is important, but is it really so time-sensitive that we can't take 30 minutes to feed our body that keeps going day in and day out?

Now stop and really think about that.

The Hunger Cycle Mindset

I'm intrigued when I watch judges in action. On the bench, they listen to the facts, straight-faced and emotionless. It's their job to listen and analyze the facts and evidence based on the law. Like these judges, you're going to use the "evidence" you *objectively observed* about your weight, diet and activity to learn where you can make improvements – not to feel bad or overly confident.

The goal is to analyze and question your data to make adjustments, changes, and decisions based on your goals and your body's needs. If the diet-monsters start to haunt your thoughts – push them away. Quiet your brain with this thought:

"When I eat, I am analyzing what's on my plate and how I feel before and after I eat. It's not about being on or off a diet. I'm learning what works best for ME."

Mastery Step

- Make a list of "trigger foods" and remove them from where they tempt you most (e.g., your house, office, car, etc.).
- Analyze the content of your meals. Do your meals include a protein, vegetables and small amount of starchy carbs?
- Stabilize the frequency of your meals. Do not let more than three to four hours lapse between meals or snacks.
- Record how you are feeling before and after meals and snacks. Hungry? Low? Energy? Craving?

CHAPTER 5

To Eat or Not to Eat

One cannot think well, love well, sleep well,
if one hasn't dined well.

– VIRGINIA WOOLF

E motions often play a big role in the choices we make in life, including when, where, and how much we eat. But emotions are meant to be felt, not fed. Eating issues may arise when we confuse emotional hunger with real hunger. This chapter is about paying close attention to your emotions in regard to your eating habits and your relationship to your body and your life.

You will practice how to pay attention to and acknowledge what you're feeling *before* you eat, and then wait just a moment before you start eating. In this way, we can identify when we are eating because we are listening to the hunger cycle or when we are eating for emotional reasons.

Physical hunger starts in the stomach, not the head. So for starters, you need to know where your stomach is located. Feel where the soft space begins between the two sides of your rib cage. Your stomach is located just slightly to the left of that space. This is where gnawing and growling starts when you are experiencing real, physical hunger. If you feel grumbling around or below your belly button, it probably has little to do with hunger. This is your small intestine doing digestive work. Most likely it's a sign that you have to pass gas or move your bowels.

Your stomach is made of muscles that expand and contract to digest your food and start it moving through your body's digestive system. When your stomach is empty, it can create quite a bit of noise. A noisy stomach is one of the first physical responses to hunger. The hydrochloric acid in your stomach may even create a slight burning feeling or pang when your stomach is empty and your hunger is real.

Physical hunger also builds gradually and is open to a variety of foods. It's usually pretty patient, unless you've waited too long and now have a flood of ghrelin hormone screaming at your brain to eat.

Emotions have nothing to do with real, physical hunger. When some people are physically hungry, they experience slight headaches or feel shaky because their blood sugar becomes low. Others get downright irritable – or "hangry," the new term for feeling angry because you're hungry.

Emotional hunger usually craves something specific like sweets or fatty carb combinations like chocolate or pizza. When we go for the craving that our mind inspires, our minds think they are feeding our bodies, but at this point the body and the mind are disconnected.

People can eat mindlessly for reasons that include boredom, fatigue, procrastination and anxiety. None of these will make your stomach growl. And eating properly may even reduce anxiety!

Sometimes when we think we're hungry, we are actually thirsty. Dehydration makes us tired or lethargic. Other times, the foods we are eating are not actually giving us energy and no matter how much of them we eat, we will still feel tired.

Happiness, sadness, loneliness, anxiety and boredom are just a few of the many emotions that can drive our eating. A telltale sign that we're eating to fulfill emotional hunger is the splash of guilt that follows the eating event. Guilt and remorse about eating are virtually non-existent when we eat to nourish our bodies.

The chart below illustrates the difference between the two types of hunger.

Physical Hunger	Emotional Hunger
"Oh, that was my stomach making those noises."	*"I need a little something sweet. Nah, an apple won't do it. Maybe something with a little chocolate."*
"I'm not sure what I want for dinner. I'm pretty open to just about anything."	*"I'm SO glad it's Friday. I've been SO good on my diet, I deserve something REALLY good to eat."*
"Mmmm. My dinner was good. I'm feeling full now."	
"Hmm ... I'm starting to get a bit hungry. I wonder what's for dinner?"	*"Uh-oh ... There's none left? I can't believe I ate that much. Why did I do that?"*
	"Oooh, that looks good. I know I shouldn't, but what the hell."

Years of dieting, grazing, overeating and bingeing have left many of us confused and out of touch with the rhythm of our body's hunger cycle. Surgical weight-loss procedures like gastric bypass and sleeve gastrectomy also interrupt the natural hunger rhythm for a short while after surgery. If you are struggling to identify whether you are actually hungry, don't worry. You are not alone.

But if you follow the three laws of My Hungry Head, with a little practice, you'll get back to your senses, literally, and begin making food choices with your body and not your feelings.

First Law: DO NOT Skip Meals

You cannot calm your Hungry Head if you haven't satisfied your hungry body. Missing meals or waiting more than four hours to eat allows ghrelin to continue building. The more ghrelin communicating with your brain, the more likely you will overeat when you finally have your meal.

Plan to wait no more than three to four hours between meals. If you have had weight-loss surgery, you may have to eat small meals every two to three hours for the first few months. Be careful not to slip into the habit of eating every hour or less. That is GRAZING, and it will lead to consuming more food than your body needs – with limited feelings of satiety.

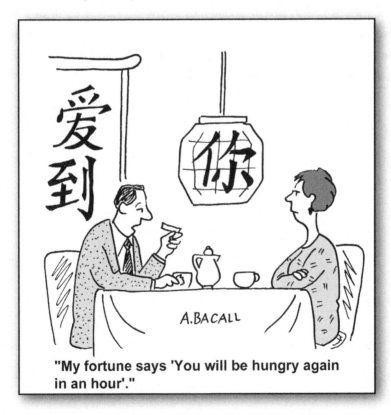

"My fortune says 'You will be hungry again in an hour'."

Eat balanced meals that include solid protein such as meat, fish, cheese or tofu; vegetables; and, if desired, a small amount of starchy carbs. This will ensure your body gets the energy and nutrients it needs to help you feel energetic and alive. Eat your protein first. Solid proteins like meat, poultry and fish make your digestive muscles work. Remember, each contraction of these muscles helps release the "I've had enough" hormones that allow your brain to register a satisfied feeling. Thirst can sometimes be mistaken for hunger, so be sure to drink enough non-caffeinated fluids.

You will not know what your body needs unless you pay attention to it. After you eat, sense how you feel immediately after, then an hour after, and then two hours after. In addition to weight-loss surgery, there are some drugs and prescription medications that affect hunger by either suppressing or stimulating appetite. If you think this may be happening to you, check with your health-care provider or pharmacist.

Second Law: Feel Your Emotions, Don't Feed Them

It is possible that you may not even recognize that you are having an emotional response when you reach for food. You may be wondering, how do I know the difference between real hunger and emotional eating?

For starters, check to see how long it has been since you last ate. Before each meal, you can also practice asking yourself how you are feeling. If you find yourself reaching for a snack that is not in your plan, ask yourself how you are feeling. Literally ask yourself out loud: "Hey self, how are you feeling right now?" and then wait for an answer. It will seem weird and awkward, but it works. If your answer does not include body hunger sensations, chances are it's your hungry head that wants to be fed.

It takes a keen sense of awareness to manage your eating patterns if you are challenged with stress, anxiety or depression. Mood often play tricks on the hungry head. For example, physical hunger and anxiety share many symptoms. Timing your meals and eating events will help you identify whether you're feeling your emotions or eating them. This can be tricky because symptoms of physical and emotional hunger may overlap. This chart shows how.

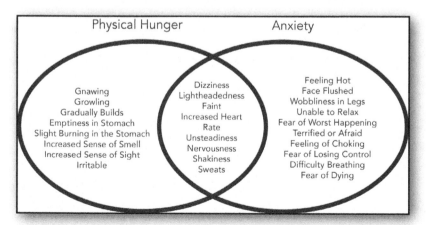

If your answer is an emotion, what are you going to do? You can quietly spend a few minutes moving your thoughts to something other than food. Unlike real hunger, emotions dissipate. Chapter 8, *Fixing the Right Problem*, offers more suggestions.

Third Law: Get Back to Your Senses – All Five of Them

To sense hunger, to sense fullness, try sensing your food. Slow down enough to let your body's communicators do their job. Food is meant to be smelled, chewed and tasted. Take your time to do this by sitting down in a calm environment to enjoy your meals, if you can. Take your time, and let your brain "hear" the messages your body sends.

Mindfulness has become a buzzword of the 21st century. There's a sea of articles in magazines, blogs and social media about mindful eating. You can go to workshops, training and retreats to practice eating mindfully. Essentially, any mindful practice brings us into the moment by bringing our attention (our minds) to the moment. If we travel at the speed of awareness, this means slowing down so that we can use all of our senses to experience what is happening. The Laws of My Hungry Head are mindful practices. Ultimately, the ability to sense *real* hunger is a mindfulness practice.

However, there is just so much you can do with mindfulness.

If you are eating food that is not nutritionally satisfying your hunger or foods that are triggering your desire to eat more, it does not matter how mindful you are. Your body will be left craving more.

Follow the My Hungry Head Laws in sequence. Satisfy your body's nutritional needs. Feed your body, not your emotions. Eat mindfully and intentionally.

In the beginning, practicing these laws may require more of your energy and attention. As you get more skilled at eating satisfying meals, feeling your emotions as they arise, and sensing your body's cues, following the My Hungry Head Laws will be a cinch.

Donna's Story

Donna, 45, a freelance writer and mother of two teens, came to my class as a professional dieter. She started her first diet when she was just 10 years old. Maybe they have diet prisons for juveniles as well as adults.

"Oh my gosh," she said when she started the My Hungry Head program. "I've lost and gained probably 50 pounds four, five, six times. I started when I was 10, doing Weight Watchers with my mom, and I've been on some kind of diet program ever since.

"It was one December morning, I woke up and said to myself,

'OK. I'm 45 years old. For at least 35 of those years, I've been trying to lose weight.'

"I've been focused on my weight for that long, and it's not that I've done the wrong things. I'm certain I have done some wrong things, but it's not for lack of trying. I exercise. I can eat the same thing that this person over here eats, and I would gain five pounds. I've gone through all these different programs. I've seen them all – I've done programs and I've done nutritionists. I've tried restricting, cutting back, and I even tried 'moderation.' These diets, they're just not always real life."

Donna came to My Hungry Head because she heard that it wasn't just another "diet" program and because it had worked for people she knew.

After a few weeks in the program, Donna discovered that she didn't really know much about her own body. Sure, she could follow a diet. But she couldn't really figure out what her own body needed.

"Yeah, the gurgling and growling. I didn't understand my body at first. I had just had weight-loss surgery, and I think I was actually thinking it was hunger, because all I heard was bubbling and gurgling. It was my intestines – not my stomach.

"OK, I see now. I've been reacting to gas and movement in my intestines. I learned to stop eating and give my gut a break."

With a little coaching, Donna became skilled at listening to her body. But her lifestyle and emotional makeup presented a challenge. She was an academic, always thinking rather than feeling, and she rarely exercised. Still, she always had to be doing something. I encouraged her to do yoga to build body awareness. She loved nature and hiking with a camera, which she continued. This was a pivotal step in helping her understand and manage her emotional eating.

Donna finally started accepting that she's a smart, creative, busy woman. She has done so many things in her life and done them well. It just happened that managing her weight wasn't one of those things – at least not yet.

"I'm not good at throwing the ball, but I can learn. I guess I can learn this, too."

Being able to identify her real hunger signs was important for Donna. "I think that's huge because I'll be honest, I've always considered it a weakness."

Donna's immediate challenge was her work situation. "I work at home, so I make my own schedule," she said. "That's sometimes a good and a bad thing, because the kitchen's always right there. I have said, I'll plan, I'll get out, go for a walk. And then usually, once I do that, it's like a reset button. In other words, once I do something healthy, I'll continue with the healthy trend.

"In theory, that often works. In practice, not always. But when I'm in the house, that's really when I have to concentrate. I have literally read a stressful email, turned around, and I'm in the kitchen. I've gone from my office and I'm in the kitchen and I'm like, 'Oh my God, how did I get here?'

"If someone had asked, 'Do you stress-eat?' I'd have said, 'No, I don't stress-eat.' After working through the My Hungry Head program, I've learned, yeah, I guess I do.

"I've learned to stop *thinking* about my body and just *listen* to what it's saying to me. I can finally hear hunger. I'm learning to feel full – and I'm learning to feel empty and know that's OK. I don't have to feed every emotion I feel. I guess the biggest thing I've learned is that nothing is going to happen if I feel my emotions. Usually they just go away if I don't entertain them. I've never learned that on ANY diet!"

For the first time in her life, Donna is no longer on a diet. She has maintained an 80-pound weight loss for more than two years.

Food Critic Exercise

I love watching the Food Network. One of my favorite shows is *Chopped*. The judges are not only master chefs, but also masters at mindful eating, at least on the show.

Here's a fun way to practice both slowing down and activating your senses. Pick any meal – breakfast, lunch or dinner – and pretend you're a famous critic on the Food Network. Now practice writing a description of your meal.

1. *Describe what you SEE on your plate. Look at details like the colors, shapes, and the way your food looks on your plate.*

_____

_____

_____

_____

_____

_____

_____

2. *Put a bite of food on your fork. SMELL it. Describe the aroma. Is it strong or weak? Sweet or floral? Foul or yummy?*

_____

_____

_____

_____

_____

_____

_____

3. *Now take a bite. What does the texture FEEL like? Is it dry? Moist? Crunchy or chewy? Soft or brittle?*

_____

_____

_____

_____

_____

_____

_____

4. *Chew slowly. What does it TASTE like? Is it sweet or salty? Acidic? Syrupy or tart?*

_____

_____

_____

_____

_____

_____

_____

Remember, you only get to taste your food while it's in your mouth, so ENJOY every bite!

To Eat or Not to Eat Mindset

Emotions are much like a sunny day at the beach. With just enough exposure, they can warm our hearts. Too much and they can scorch our souls. Another way to think about emotions is to view them like a running river. If a river flows into a dam, a pool of water will accumulate. Too much water and a rush of rapids flows over the dam. Riverbank's too high? You may get a deep, mucky body of water. If the bank's too low, you may have a shallow brook.

Think about your emotions. Do you hold on to your feelings until they overflow like a river over a dam? Do you ignore them and feel stuck in murky waters where you no longer know what you're feeling? Or perhaps you're constantly expressing emotions with little depth in other areas of your life.

Emotions are a wonderful and powerful part of being human. They can play a big role in the choices we make in life, including when, where and how much we eat. But emotions are meant to be felt, not fed. Problems begin when we confuse emotional hunger with real hunger. Quiet your brain with this thought:

*"I am feeling my emotions, not feeding them. I'm listening to my body's physical cues before and after my meals
and learning to SENSE what I am feeling and eating."*

Mastery Step

- Identify whether your hunger is physical or emotional.
- Feel your feelings – they will go away if you don't entertain them or feed them.
- Practice the food critic exercise each time you eat. Engage your senses when you eat. Use your sight, taste, smell and touch to be in the moment, rather than lost in an emotion.

CHAPTER 6

Retrain Your Brain

No matter what it is, I can have enough.
I can have more later.

— MB SHERRIN

When I was in my mid-20s, I tried my hand at six-on-six volleyball. I looked forward to weekly pickup games at our local YMCA. Although I was new to the game, I enjoyed the competition. There were a few other beginners, but most of the players were at the intermediate level, with the exception of one guy, Dominik, who had competed on Poland's men's indoor team for the Olympics.

I thought I had hit the coaching jackpot. I would learn all I could from the Olympian, then dominate my YMCA competitors. When I mustered up the courage to ask Dominik how I could learn to play competitively, he told me, "It's too late. You'll never be able to play well. You're too old."

Years later, when I felt myself losing my battle with the scale, I would think about Dominik. I knew my weight problem was mostly in my head, and I already sensed that I would need to change deeply ingrained habits. Could I ever learn to eat with a sense of control and freedom from guilt? Was I too old to learn this new skill?

Happily for me and hopefully for you, it turned out that I was able to learn it. With My Hungry Head program, there's no need to flounder around the volleyball court of life.

You might finally be eating high-quality foods. You've stopped skipping meals and you've developed a regular eating schedule. But you struggle to control the urge to eat more. You're still mindlessly reaching for second helpings. Or the will to continue walking past your co-worker's candy dish is fading. It may feel like an unruly teenager is living rent-free in your head.

It's possible to calm your inner dialogue. To see that this is a hard, but winnable struggle, let's look at how three of my clients did it.

Brenda

Brenda had been heavy her entire life. Not a day went by when she wasn't embarrassed about her weight or afraid to try something new.

"Even after weight-loss surgery," she said, "I knew I still had more work to do. I had to fix my head.

"It was really weird at first, but it worked. I tell people who have unsuccessfully tried to lose weight and keep it off that the process of calming my head around food was the most effective learning tool."

Success didn't come easily. It took some time for her to believe "That was good. I've had enough. I can have more later."

"In the past," she said, "when I was at a restaurant, it would be like, 'Oh my God. This is so good. I can't leave that.' And I'd eat it anyway, even if I was full. Now I talk myself through it: 'Yes, I can stop now. I can leave food on my plate. I really can have more later. Maybe not tomorrow, but nobody's stopping me from coming back and having it again.'"

Brenda lost nearly 100 pounds and is virtually guilt-free. She no longer thinks "ice cream" and suddenly finds herself at Dairy Queen, devouring an entire creamy Blizzard.

In the past, she said, "I just couldn't do the things that my brain and soul wanted to do. I'd dream of going zip-lining. Now, I do. I tried canoeing and didn't have to worry about not fitting into the canoe. I'm not embarrassed to be in front of people. I'm more outgoing. It's practice. It's work. But the results have been amazing."

Judy

After having gastric bypass surgery, Judy had little trouble controlling her weight. Low levels of ghrelin left her with very little appetite.

"I was on cloud nine," she recalls after decreasing the weight on her 5-foot frame from 197 pounds to 128.

But when the honeymoon ended, Judy quickly regained 20 pounds. She knew she had to learn new weight-control skills fast.

For Judy, the key was "figuring out if I was eating to stuff down my emotions. In the past, I was trying to eat as much as I could to fill an emotional hole. I just didn't want to feel my feelings anymore."

After gastric bypass surgery, she couldn't stuff her smaller stomach without painful consequences. "For so long, I was confused about my body's cues. I had to actually come face to face with my emotions and feelings."

Understanding the physiological hunger cycle brought some calm and order to Judy's thinking.

"Now I look at food differently. It's there to nourish me, to fuel me and to do good things for my body. It doesn't take away any of the pain or the hurt feelings I was having."

At the same time, Judy was slowly developing new coping skills to deal with day-to-day issues.

"I constantly remind myself I don't have to solve all of my problems in one day. I have a deeper understanding of what's important and what's not."

One skill that Judy learned to employ well was choosing to do NOTHING. Pausing instead of reacting has made a world of difference.

"I remind myself all the time, 'I'm fine.' I can just breathe the air and feel a sense of peace. I had to work more on my soul, which has helped to complete – or fill – me more."

Judy grew up thinking of food as love.

"Now I know there's so much more that can be love," she says. "I have strong faith and I'm learning more about who I am as a person and what I need to get by day-to-day. I know it's so much more than just food."

Melinda

Melinda came to me with the sole purpose of maintaining the 130-pound weight loss she had achieved after gastric bypass surgery four years ago. She was driven by a fear that the weight would return if she didn't fix what caused her to gain weight in the first place. She feared that she was slowly edging back to old habits, the ones that caused to her to eat more after every diet. A true culinary recidivist. "In my brain, I can hear a voice that says 'You'd better eat it. Who knows when you're gonna have it again?"

She feared that when she took a proactive approach to limiting portions, the reruns of the clean-plate club would return: "Throw it out? Are you kidding?! You can't waste it. You'd better eat it."

After repeating the My Hungry Head mantra – *That was good. I've had enough. I can have more later.* – Melinda started to believe it.

"I've dieted for so many years and I've never heard that before. I've said it to myself thousands of times since. It's a game-changer for me."

For Melinda, this mind exercise eliminates the fear of deprivation. "I don't have to shovel food in because I don't know when I'm gonna get it again. It's like having the holiday-food mentality: 'I'd better eat lots. Who knows if I'll have turkey again until next year."

With a bit of practice, Melinda was able to really believe that apple pie is available all year – she doesn't have to gorge at Thanksgiving or any other day, for that matter!

At this stage of Melinda's journey, she began accepting that there was no scarcity of the foods on which she had once binged.

"I stopped feeling like I can never have something I like again, even if it is something seasonal. When I tell myself, 'I've had enough, I can have more later,' it gives me permission to believe the future is OK. It's not going to be a future of deprivation."

She continued to work on quieting the old voices in her head, too. Some of them were from childhood: "You have to eat everything on your plate. There are people starving everywhere."

"Now I know that's just someone else's rule that I no longer have to live by or react to," she said. Changing her childhood messages hasn't been easy, she said, "but I do it."

Rather than clean the plate, "I'll save it and eat it next time. No more 'someone is starving somewhere' excuse. I'm not solving world hunger by eating more. And I'm not starving anymore. This is a huge change to my mindset."

Melinda didn't want to be told what to do. She wanted a process that addressed her life – her thoughts. After years of dieting and a net gain of 150 pounds, Melinda proved to herself that diet programs weren't giving her lasting results. Her process through My Hungry Head confirmed that the struggle is real and that it's OK.

"Knowing there was a no-judgment zone was a key difference. Knowing I could say, 'I'm struggling' and hear someone say 'I overeat, too. Now where do we go from here? How do we not eat that bag of Fritos next time?' Taking away the rules and deprivation has made all the difference."

The Voices in Our Heads

I've never thought of Sigmund Freud as a weight-control guru, but the father of psychoanalysis may have had something to contribute in this area.

Freud considered personality a dynamic interaction between what he called the id, the ego, and the superego. I like to think of the id as the pleasure-seeking wild child. On the other hand, the superego is all about doing things "right." It's our conscience, or the little angel on our shoulder that says "don't do it." Stuck in the middle is the ego, the voice of reason.

The ego, or adult voice, is seldom heard within those of us struggling with chronic on-again, off-again dieting. Our goodie-two-shoes superego is hell-bent on following the rules, counting every calorie and planning to exercise *every day*. And there's our wild-child id rebelling, flipping off the super-ego while partaking of a pile of cheesy nachos.

If we want to tame our hungry head, our adult voice has to speak up. This whole process may be unconscious to you initially, but as soon as you recognize it, there is no going back. You can consciously take the reins by giving your adult voice, your ego, a place at the table.

Your Hungry Head wants to hear an adult voice – YOUR voice.

The turning point in calming your Hungry Head is to take the reins and tell yourself and your goody-two-shoes angel that it's OK to eat when you are hungry. Tell the diet-angel that it is not only OK, but also crucial that you enjoy your food. Then let your wild-child id know that you've *had ENOUGH and you can have more later.*

Part of calming your hungry head is letting go of judgment and guilt that has built up through years of negative diet experiences. You don't have a weak or flawed character just because diets haven't worked to maintain weight loss. There's much more to it than that.

Your body has an intricate wiring system that influences how we think and act. Electrical impulses travel throughout our bodies along these wires, making thoughts and behaviors happen. The more that an impulse travels along a certain path, the faster your response. The same message, or behavior, over and over will get you a fast response without a second thought.

When I teach My Hungry Head workshops, I often use the analogy of a snowy mountain. As the snowcapped mountain warms, melted water begins a journey downward. More and more water will flow toward the path of least resistance. Consecutive drops of water carve a deeper and deeper path down the mountain. A drop becomes a stream. A stream becomes a river. With enough snow melting, a gentle stream turns into roaring rapids.

Thoughts – negative or positive – behave like melting water down a mountain. Messages we send ourselves about being on a diet and off a diet run through our neurological systems. A history of chronic dieting and the negative messages attached to every rebound pound act like river rapids in our brains.

Need proof? How do you feel when you hear "bathing suit weather is coming"? It's no surprise that this simple phrase can send shivers down the spine of a serial dieter in a split second.

And we can't discount the powerful system reinforcing the messages in our hungry heads. It is estimated that the fast-food industry spends up to $4.2 billion yearly on advertising. And the messages start early, with children viewing up to 13 fast-food TV advertisements daily.

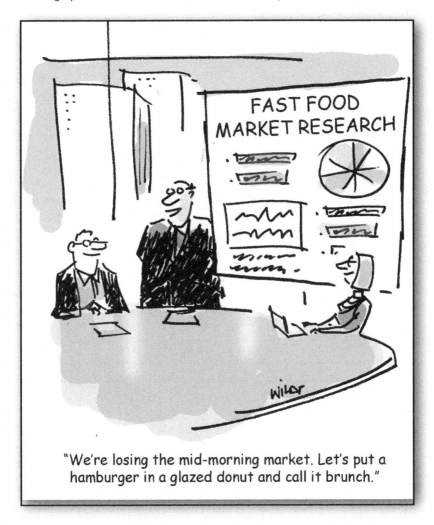

"We're losing the mid-morning market. Let's put a hamburger in a glazed donut and call it brunch."

Our senses are assaulted daily with stylized ads suggesting that McDonald's can get us lovin' life with a juicy burger or that we'll be more effective if we Run on-Dunkin'. Never in the history of mankind have calorie-dense, nutritionally deficient foods been so readily available. Our wild-child id is surrounded by temptation.

Calming Inner Dialogue

How do we change the automatic thoughts and behaviors that cause us to overindulge? How do we create new thoughts and behaviors that help us have a better relationship with food, with our bodies and with our lives?

1. Start by enjoying your food. Pay attention. Actually say the words "That was good." This will help your brain register that you actually ate.
2. Stop eating after you finish an appropriate portion. Stop *before* you feel full. Then say "I've had ENOUGH."
3. 3. When you are done, quietly and convincingly, tell yourself: "I can have MORE LATER."

These three simple messages yielded profound results in my life. My body and my mind were finally present when I ate. I actually started to believe that ENOUGH was OK. And knowing that I could have MORE LATER calmed the desperate dieter in me.

Top athletes and musicians know something that can help people struggling with eating difficulties.

Athletes practice over and over and over in order to master their sport. Musicians practice over and over and over to play beautiful music.

People who achieve success with My Hungry Head practice the tools over and over and over. Every day and every meal are opportunities to practice. There's no magic bullet. There's no easy way to the Olympics or Carnegie Hall. Practice, repetition and paying attention are what's going to calm your Hungry Head.

Retrain Your Brain Mindset

Imagine you're a little kid who is told no every time you want to play or when you ask to have what the other kids have. Picture trying to understand why foods that taste so good are so bad. Recall how advertising and media machines tell us to eat more and lose weight all at the same time. Is it any wonder that we feel anxious or overwhelmed?

Sure, we all need to live within boundaries and rules. But what about enjoyment, fun and satisfaction? After years of on-again, off-again dieting, our brains are confused. Now it's time to settle your brain's conflicting desires to eat more and weigh less with calming adult-like messages.

The Retrain Your Brain Mindset is about doing the work necessary to build a positive network of messages that calm the impulsive and critical voices in your head. Quiet your brain with this thought:

"Like an athlete or musician, I am building an effective, positive network of messages to calm the impulsive and critical voices in my head."

Mastery Step

- Be sure to eat three meals. Do not wait more than three to four hours to eat. Remember, you will not be able to calm your hungry head if you don't feed your hungry body!
- Use planned snacks if you need to or want to.
- Repeat after every meal and snack: "That was good. I've had enough. I can have more later."

CHAPTER 7

Living Between Meals

> We clean our plates, yet we're still famished –
> starving for something other than food.
>
> – KATE WICKER

M anaging your weight is not just about eating. It's also about what you do when you're NOT eating. How you live life between meals will have a significant impact on the weight you lose and keep off. Generating new ideas and approaches to emotional eating will be our focus.

Much of your success will revolve around how you use time. Do you take enough time to follow My Hungry Head practices? Or do you seem to have so much time that you fill it with mindless eating?

Yes, managing a healthy weight takes time and effort. We are not just talking about practicing the My Hungry Head process here, but also taking time to make the kinds of meals that work, taking time to move your body, taking time to be mindful of what you are doing.

All too often I hear patients complain they don't have enough time to eat well or to move their bodies. After further discussion, I usually learn that they don't like cooking or going to the gym. Watching prime-time crime shows always wins out. Time actually has nothing to do with it.

Many people do, indeed, have demanding and stressful jobs. But I've met few who can't work more efficiently and save a little extra time for healthy practices. We tend to find time for what's really important to us.

By taking time to do something that sustains us and feeds us on a deeper level, we actually end up feeling like we have more time! In many ways, it comes down to choice. We all have 24 hours each day. How are you spending your time?

Make an honest assessment of what you do each day and how much of what you do either feeds your life or depletes it. Track your use of time for a week. You can do this from memory or actually take a week to explore this. Use your objective observer skills. No judgment.

What does the rhythm of your day look like? Is there any time left over? Is every waking moment filled? Do you get at least six to eight hours of sleep? Remember that lack of sleep lowers levels of the hormone leptin, which signals when you have had enough to eat. What about TV or computer time? Is it more than an hour or two?

How you use your 24 hours will have a significant impact on your ability to manage your weight.

What's Happening?

As you consider the evidence you've gathered, ask yourself what's happening with your time? What is the balance between work, play and "down" time? Did you notice any trends?

Are you skipping steps in the My Hungry Head program because you feel you don't have time to prepare for success? Are you doing too much? What is your perceived stress level? Are you so stressed that you aren't even aware of the choices you're making?

Or is life pretty quiet ... perhaps TOO quiet? Did you notice a pattern of boredom or evening TV, complete with mindless snacking?

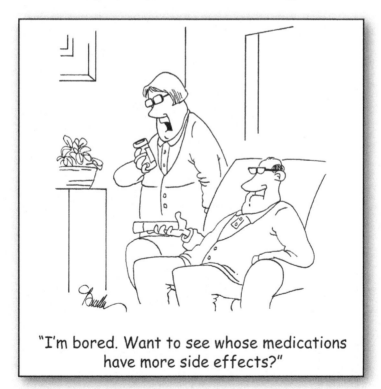

"I'm bored. Want to see whose medications have more side effects?"

A word here about watching television and other visual/media stimulation. Often we fool ourselves into thinking that sitting back on the couch and watching TV is our "down time" in the same way that we can fool ourselves by saying we deserve that treat on Friday afternoon after a long week at work. It may be that an hour on the couch watching one show or playing a video game for an hour can be down time, but three or four hours? In the end, you are probably not rewarding yourself.

Most people struggling with a hungry head fall into one of the following categories in terms of time. Which one of these sounds the most like you? After we identify that, we can concentrate on generating ideas to better use our time.

Unfocused

Preparation takes time. It can be your time OR someone else's. You may need to schedule time to practice the My Hungry Head program or get some help from someone in your life to prepare meals and snacks for you.

What can you eliminate from your day to make time for preparation?

Is there anyone who can help you prepare? Cook your meals? Make your lunch?

Are there any shortcuts you're willing to try? Maybe a meal-sharing group or healthy precooked foods?

Stressed Out

Ask yourself this question: Am I doing too many things that I *must* do OR is that I am not able to say *NO* to certain things or people in my life?

If you want to lose weight and keep if off, there's no way around it – you have to make some hungry head time. Making things as simple for yourself as possible is important when you are learning new skills and changing habits.

Try this: Imagine you are only allowed to do THREE things each day. What will you say "YES" to? What will you say "NO" to?

If you are not good at saying "no," you are not alone. Sometimes making yourself a priority feels selfish. Imagine that you are saying "yes" to yourself, your health, and your life. Practice gentle ways of saying "no," like "I'd love to, but I can't right now." Or "Sure, I'd love to help, but I can't this week. How about next week?"

Don't kid yourself, this is a hard exercise, especially for those of us who pride ourselves on being responsible, caring people!

You may need a friend, health coach or someone with an objective point of view to help you through this exercise.

Bored

Boredom is a common ingredient in creating a Hungry Head. It's time for an activity makeover if you're finding yourself eating mindlessly in front of the television or opening the refrigerator door over and over, hoping for a tasty new snack to miraculously appear.

Challenge yourself to list 10 things you would enjoy doing that DO NOT involve food. The key here is to list things you'll ENJOY doing! If you LOVE to clean your house or do laundry, then put it on the list. Otherwise, focus on enjoyable things you'd like to do. Maybe there are things you wish you could do, but feel you need to wait to lose weight to do them. Put them on the list, too, and start doing them anyway.

There are so many other things you can do for "down time." Maybe they are activities that you would put on the enjoyable list, maybe not. Some ideas are: read a book, go for a walk in nature, take a nap, call a friend for a nice chat, meditate, knit. What other down-time ideas can you come up with? Down time should give you a chance to rest your body and your mind and leave you feeling refreshed and ready for work and the activities you enjoy doing.

The Chemistry of Being Alive

In his book *The Power of Myth*, Joseph Campbell says, "People say that what we're all seeking is a meaning for life. I don't think that's what we're really seeking. I think that what we're seeking is an experience of being alive."

So what does it mean, literally, to be alive? We can look to our brains for one way to answer this question.

Here is a guided tour of brain hormones that affect how you feel and perhaps how you eat. If it includes more detail than you want, feel free to skip directly to the Mastery Step at the end of the chapter.

The brain is a three-pound collection of nerve tissue that processes information and helps us makes sense of the world. Included are several important molecules that influence our feelings and emotions – or "happy brain" molecules. These include GABA, oxytocin, adrenaline, serotonin, endocannabinoids, endorphins and dopamine. Understanding how these neurological gems work in our own brains may provide clues in helping us enjoy more productive, binge-free time between meals.

Stressed or Anxious?

GABA and oxytocin play key roles in creating a sense of well-being. GABA helps to slow nerves from firing – calming an overexcited nervous system. Oxytocin has earned a reputation as the "cuddle hormone." Studies have shown that intimacy, such as touch, hugs, cuddling and spending time in groups, naturally increases oxytocin. It also increases after spending time with animals. If you're single and have no furry friends available, you can effectively calm an excited nervous system by meditating or practicing yoga.

Chronic Pain Got You Down?

Looking for a blissful, pain-free feeling? Endocannabinoids and endorphins are the main players here. It was once thought that "runner's high" was associated with increased endorphins, but it seems that endocannabinoids have more to do with the "bliss" feeling. Aerobic activities such as distance running, hiking and long walks are closely associated with increases in endocannabinoids, while physical exertion and anaerobic activities such as sprinting, weightlifting and orgasm (vs. cuddling) are more aligned with the pain-free, feel-good endorphin chemicals.

Hope and Confidence

Substances such as sugar, alcohol and drugs used excessively have been implicated in stimulating reward-sensitive chemicals like dopamine in our brain. Dopamine has a reputation as the reward chemical because it appears to increase with the anticipation of something positive. Discovering new things, creating to-do lists and setting goals also have a positive impact on dopamine without the negative consequences of abusing substances like sugar, alcohol and drugs. The sense of accomplishment that comes with achieving a goal or completing a task has a positive effect on serotonin. Even making a list of your strengths bumps up this feel-good chemical. All this equates to less impetus to "stress-eat."

Energy & Focus

Caffeine is the most widely used legal drug in America. Why? Because it helps people focus. It comes with a price, though. Its effect is short-lived, creating a vicious cycle of needing more and more. It can also be a pesky stomach irritant, especially for those who have had weight-loss surgery. If you are sick of the couch potato feeling or you're lacking the focus to start or stick with an activity or task, a short burst of high-intensity exercise may give you the shot of adrenaline you need. Don't overcomplicate things with unachievable workout schedules. And there's no need to run a marathon – unless you want to. Your brain – and stomach – will thank you.

Not all the happy chemicals will align at once, but with the right activities, your brain can change over time. And so will you.

Mike's Story

When Mike joined the My Hungry Head program, he was 33 years old and weighed 683 pounds. He's not sure whether this was his highest weight, because he didn't have access to a scale that registered more than 500 pounds.

Mike always struggled with his weight ("I was a big kid most of my life"), but the problem really got out of hand in his 20s. "I was always overweight, but I was functional," he said. "Then the weight got to a point where I couldn't bring the trash to the street corner without having to take a break."

A series of life challenges left Mike in full retreat. He was unemployed and living with his parents. His once-active social life faded away after each invitation he refused or ignored.

"The worst part of my weight was that it killed me socially. I love hosting parties and attending social functions. I shut down and I lost all of my friends. I just stopped hanging out with them. I felt like a hindrance." He had a profound fear of dying, "but I wasn't living, either."

Mike wouldn't qualify as a candidate for safe weight-loss surgery until he lost nearly 150 pounds. Over the next six months, he would spend each week in our classes, working the program and talking with others who shared the same struggle.

"It's easier to be in a group with people who get it," he said. "It bugs me when I hear someone that weighs 200 pounds consider themselves overweight. It's like ... 'Oh, yeah, you're wicked overweight, buddy. You're at my goal weight.' Sure, he could lose some weight, but he doesn't know my struggle. He doesn't know what it's like to walk through a grocery store and have a little kid point to you and go, 'Look, Mom, he's huge.'"

Mike, a stand-up comic, joked, "I can't punch a little kid. You know it's frowned upon. So I walk by and whisper, 'Santa's not real.' It's my only revenge."

On the surface, his joke is funny. Underneath, there's a sadness.

This wasn't Mike's first time at the weight-loss rodeo. "I've lost weight before. I know how to do it. It's staying with it when you're down and struggling that's the hard part."

The process of setting goals and spending time with a group of people began to change the course of Mike's weight-loss journey. "When I'm around people that know, that have the same struggles and the same journey, it just makes it easier. I'm not sticking out. I can feel like a person."

He lost more than 100 pounds before weight-loss surgery. Nearly a year later, he lost an additional 170 pounds after gastric sleeve surgery. Mike continues to lose weight in small, regular increments as he limits his portions and continues to find activities he enjoys. "Figuring out what I want to do with my life seems to have helped the most," he said.

Mike excels at generating meaningful ways to live between meals. He's now doing stand-up comedy – a longtime goal. He enjoys high-intensity workouts balanced with meditation in a serene park by the ocean. "I'm lovin' life now. I have my routines, I'm focused, and I know what I want to do with my life. Next on life's agenda – seriously – is skydiving and swimming with sharks."

Living Between Meals Mindset

What you do with your time between meals is just as important as what you eat. I've seen hundreds of books and lists of "100 Things to Do Instead of Eating." Some people benefit from these resources, but most don't. Why? Because it's not THEIR list.

Living successfully between meals is as individual as what you put on your plate. The Living Between Meals Mindset is about generating possibilities, NOT barriers or excuses. It's the willingness to look inward and discover what is really important to you, then growing a list of new ideas – without criticizing or evaluating them. Quiet your brain with this thought:

"I am finding new ways to live between meals that make sense for me. I'm open to discovering new ideas, possibilities and alternatives."

Mastery Step

- What's important to me that doesn't involve food?
- What do I love to do, want to do, dream about having in my life?
- Having difficulty preparing for success? Generate 10 ideas that would help you prepare to make better choices to manage your weight.
- Pressed for time because you're doing too much? Generate a list of 10 things to which you're willing to say "no" or "not right now."
- Too much time on your hands? Does boredom have the better of you? Make a list of 10 things you would like to do that DO NOT involve food.

Place your list where you need to see it most (e.g., on the refrigerator, snack cabinet, bathroom mirror, etc.). Your mindset for practice is to no longer let those five words –"I do not have time"– stand between you and success.

CHAPTER 8

Fixing the Right Problem

> *We can't solve problems using the same kind of*
> *thinking we used to create them.*
>
> – ALBERT EINSTEIN

B y now, you are probably getting a sense that there's much more to managing weight than just eating less and exercising more. With the diet prison, there's no "get out of jail free" card. Managing stress is one critical component in calming your hungry head.

Identifying the underlying problems that get you off-track is no easy task. It's easy to blame and complain, but where did that ever get you?

I'm guilty of this, too. I remember that every diet I tried would start with hope and excitement. Inevitably, I'd find some reason why I couldn't stick to it. I couldn't see myself eating off-the-shelf boxed foods while my family ate freshly cooked meals. I loved food too much to live on shakes just to lose a few pounds. And I was also done forking over membership dues to my local gym. I'd had it with detailed exercise programs, sodium-laden frozen dinners, and showing up for weigh-ins that felt like more like shame-ins, all while striving to reach a goal I wasn't sure was even right for me.

My personal journey of calming my hungry head improved significantly when I took a big step back and looked at my own life. At this point, I accepted there was no magic diet-pixie dust that would manage my weight. I had to take a critical look at how I could take care of myself in ways that made sense for me.

I've watched hundreds of weight-loss patients struggle with the same issues. Even my patients who appeared successful at weight loss admitted that they "white-knuckled" it. They tried as hard as they could to make the square diet-peg fit into the round hole – their life. They could be physically healthy, but emotionally, they were miserable. They couldn't seem to find the weight where they were both healthy *and* happy. What's more disturbing is that my patients, and millions of others, attributed this trap to their own failing – or lack of willpower.

Could it be that they're attempting to do something that just doesn't work for their lifestyle? For their values?

This chapter will take you through the process of identifying what derails your success and what maintains it. Why put lots of energy into a solution if you don't have the correct problem? This process starts with examining three areas: your basic needs, your vision of a quality life, and the obstacles in the way of the life you envision.

Are Your Basic Needs Met?

For decades, human development theorists such as Abraham Maslow and William Glasser advocated that all humans have a set of basic needs that must be met before they can develop their full potential. For example, every human must have the essentials of human life, such as food, water, shelter, good health and safety. It is the rare few who are able to overcome a lack of life's necessities.

Our hunger cycle is an intricate, undeniable system designed to keep us alive. It wants us to eat.

Our bodies crave a multitude of vitamins and minerals that we can get from food. Those who have had weight-loss surgery must accommodate for nutritional deficiencies with physician-recommended vitamin supplements. You may be able to get away with skipping a meal here or there, but make a steady habit of it and you'll find yourself pushing the proverbial rock uphill. Physiology trumps willpower. Always.

What Does a "Quality Life" Look Like to You?
Having a sense of power and freedom are also basic human needs that must be met. A sense of accomplishment, self-esteem and the ability to make choices contribute to a sense of calm in one's life.

Interestingly, many of my patients who have done exceptionally well at maintaining long-term weight loss have income at, or below, the poverty line. It seems that their core struggle was meeting basic needs – quality food and access to health care and education. Once they learned how to budget their minimal, fixed income to secure quality food, they began to feel accomplished and empowered to care for themselves and their family.

On the other hand, more often than not, I see patients with greater means adrift in a sea of choices – and not always making the best ones for themselves. And it's not limited to poor food choices. In my experience, I've seen patients manage their finances in an eerily similar way to the way they manage their weight. In my clinical practice, more than 70 percent of our patients live beyond their means.

Why the similarities between food and money? First, we need both to survive. Second, both require budgeting: We all have biological responsibilities that we must meet, just as we do financial obligations. Financial security requires budgeting. A healthy body requires a budgeting process, too. Your body needs X number of calories to survive. Eat – or spend – over your calorie limit, and your debt will appear in extra weight. From a psycho-social standpoint, food is subject to the same influences as money. There's a temptation to want more of both – and the easier it is to obtain, the better. And the magazines we read and even the music we listen to are constantly telling us that we don't have enough of either one.

So what truly makes you feel accomplished – a number on the scale? Or is it something more? Do you feel you have the ability to control your choices with food? With exercise? With other areas in your life?

The power of imagination is undeniable. Think about Winston Churchill's famous quote "You create your own universe as you go along. The stronger your imagination, the more variegated your universe. When you leave off dreaming, the universe ceases to exist." Think about how you want food to fit into your universe.

Like many people, I was raised with food at the center of our family. All seven of us sat together every night for dinner. Holidays were day-long feasts of unending Italian dishes. I cannot for a second imagine a life without gathering around food. I love that part of my life. On the other hand, and completely alien to me, my husband and his family eat to live. It would be easier to nail Jell-O to a tree than it would be to get them to sit for dinner.

One relationship with food is no better or worse than the other. Negotiating the differences is the critical step to finding what's best for you.

Pleasure and the ability to play and laugh are also part of being human and alive.

How do you see yourself eating well and enjoying life?

_____

_____

_____

_____

_____

_____

What will that look like day-to-day?

_____

_____

_____

_____

_____

_____

What are you willing to give up in order to manage your weight?

_____

_____

_____

_____

_____

_____

_____

What are you unwilling to give up?

_____

_____

_____

_____

_____

_____

Once you have an image of how you want food to fit into your life, take a step back and compare this image to what is actually happening. What's in the gap between how you want be and what is actually happening? This requires taking a bird's-eye view. Be as objective as possible. This isn't the time for criticizing, blaming, complaining or punishing yourself. It's time to take a step back and put your analytical skills to work.

What are your goals? How do you want your day-to-day "life" to be?

_____

_____

_____

_____
_____
_____
_____
_____

What is your day-to-day "life" actually like?

_____
_____
_____
_____
_____
_____

What is causing the gap?

_____
_____
_____
_____
_____
_____

What could be the root cause of the gap? Keep asking "why" until you get to the root cause.

_____
_____
_____
_____

_____

_____

_____

How can close the gap between what you want and what is actually happening? Generate as many solutions as you can. Just list the possible solutions – don't evaluate them or say they won't work. Just list them!

_____

_____

_____

_____

_____

_____

_____

_____

_____

_____

_____

_____

Now choose a solution you are willing to try – put it into practice.

One Size Doesn't Fit All

Let's meet Sarah, John and Carol. They all got the same advice from their doctors – eat less and exercise more. But it wasn't so simple for them.

Sarah, stay-at-home mom

During her last pregnancy, Sarah gained 80 pounds. She was able to lose all but 10 pounds. Juggling three kids' activities has left her running around all day with little time to prepare meals. Recently, Sarah regained six pounds since her last doctor's appointment. She is feeling increasingly anxious about regaining her weight.

Sarah loves spending time with her kids and wouldn't give it up for the world. She also wants to be sure they have good eating habits. However, prepared foods and eating on the go are the norm for her family. Relying on hot dogs, chicken nuggets and frozen dinners is convenient, but it is not teaching her kids how to eat well – nor is it helping her maintain her weight loss.

"I don t have time to shop, chop and cook every night," she says. "I have to get the kids where they need to go and chase a 2-year old."

Sarah's top priorities are managing her home and her children's activities – not following a special diet for herself. A closer look at Sarah's journals shows that her calorie intake isn't too bad, but her food quality is quite poor. A lot of salty, fatty processed food is leaving her feeling bloated and sluggish.

What do you think the real issue with Sarah is?

She wants to take care of herself, but clearly feels that she does not have enough time. What she lacks are efficient ways to create meals ahead of time. She needs to think outside the box about how to incorporate a healthier lifestyle into her busy home life.

At this point, Sarah needs new ideas that make sense for a stay-at-home mom. Learning about healthy prepared foods and some easy Crock-Pot recipes could take Sarah a long way.

Planning three to four days ahead of time and preparing snacks to have on hand for herself and her kids would help when hunger hits while she is on the run. Finding ways to exercise that include her kids would also help, as well as looking for times when she can get a break from her kids to refresh.

John, Type II diabetic

John is a senior account executive for a large high-tech firm in the city. Although he is paid very well, he finds his job unfulfilling. "It's not a horrible job. I just don't like it. It's not what I want to do with my life, but it pays the bills." Eating on the road with clients and frequent dinners out with his wife contributed to John getting diabetes.

Since he started dieting, he cut out restaurant eating and lowered his blood sugar significantly. However, John is slipping back to some old habits. He's getting bored "dieting" – eating grilled chicken and salads. His blood sugars are starting to creep up again. His journal shows him on a slippery slope, back to eating rich pasta dishes and saucy, sautéed restaurant entrees. "What am I supposed to do? Eating out is a huge part of our lives!"

So what's the real issue with John?

John and his wife love to connect over dinner. Now that they're empty-nesters, he wants to spend "quality time" with his wife. "I put up with this job all week. I deserve to spend my money doing something that makes me happy."

Sure, learning to make healthy meals together may be a good start. And taking cooking lessons together may be another good idea for spending time as a couple. But John has a deeper question to answer: Is there really a restaurant or dish that will make him feel truly "satisfied"? John made significant progress calming his hungry head when he took a step back to discover what he really wanted to do with his time – and money.

Carol, single mother

Balancing a full-time job, staying on top of two busy teenagers, and running the house is about all she can handle. Carol barely has any time left over for exercise. She has been doing great at losing weight. However, she recently hit a plateau and is starting to get very frustrated.

Homemade meals are no problem for Carol. She takes pride in learning new recipes and making sure her kids eat well. But a closer analysis of Carol's weekly activities shows five or six trips to the grocery store a week! "I don't want to eat the same thing over and over. I'll get bored."

Although it is great that she is experimenting and eager to explore with recipes, Carol's unorganized approach to menu planning is taking valuable time – and contributing to impulsive snack purchases.

What do you think would really help Carol?

Is it that she lacks dedication to exercise? Maybe, but what she tells us is that she has no time. Could she use all the time she spends shopping for ingredients that she does not have on hand to exercise? Perhaps, but the only way to find out is to free up some of that time and make it available to her.

Carol would benefit greatly from planning her menus ahead of time and organizing her lists so that she only has to shop once a week. Helping her plan better and getting her teenagers to help will limit those extra trips to the grocery store and free up some time for physical activities.

Jenna's Story

Sometimes the issues are even more complex.

Jenna had battled her weight since adolescence. She grew up in a home where there was active alcoholism and substance abuse. While her mother was consumed with managing her professional career and crises at home, Jenna was abused by her brother and father. She sought comfort in her music – and food. She was an accomplished musician and recipient of a scholarship to one of the nation's most prestigious music programs. Riddled with anxiety, though, Jenna left college and settled into an accounting clerk position.

I met Jenna just after she had lost 80 pounds. This loss brought her weight down to 296 pounds. Her 5-foot-3 frame was hurting. She was now 38 years old, medicated for high blood pressure and suffering from chronic pain due to the excessive weight on her joints. However, these challenges didn't dim her bright smile and vibrant personality.

I knew there was more to Jenna than tracking accounts – and so did she. She had a vivid image of where she could be. "I know I'm smart and I have talent. I don't know why I can't get out of my own way."

Jenna attended many of my classes. She seemed determined to get her emotional eating under control, yet for every step forward, she took two steps back. Why was this happening? Why did Jenna hit the milk and cookies every time she achieved a weight goal?

A closer look revealed Jenna's "support" was actually working against her. As her weight decreased and confidence increased, Jenna returned to school to complete her college degree. As studying replaced her party nights, her friends grew more distant. Jenna was home alone, soothing herself with school work and Oreos. Her path to success grew lonely.

"I'm surrounded by people who hate change. They get so jealous every time I start to change. I'm trying to make my life better, but it feels worse than when I started."

Jenna's real problem was two-fold. She needed to be around like-minded peers who shared her journey and respected the effort she needed to put in to achieve her goals. Over the course of a few months, Jenna developed new connections with fellow students in study groups and peer events. She also redefined her relationship with old friends. Some targeted counseling helped her work through the changing relationships with her friends and her family.

After nine years, Jenna has maintained more than 80 percent of her weight loss and completed her college degree. "I learned that food isn't always the problem. I can manage my emotional eating so much better when I'm managing the important things in my life."

Fixing the Right Problem Mindset

My favorite thing about flying is looking down and seeing an entire city in one view. Everything, from the houses and buildings to the roads and rivers, looks tiny and manageable.

Life does get hectic and filled with details – big and small. The ability to step back and take a bird's-eye view is critical to identifying the best path forward. Your journey is unique. What works for one person may not work for you. Why put lots of energy into a solution if you aren't addressing the correct problem?

Life is an improvisation. Identifying when you must take a new road and staying nimble enough to change direction are key to keeping your weight off. This mindset is about slowing down to take stock, evaluating your current situation and questioning what is really happening.

"I am stepping back to look at the big picture before starting a new plan or falling into the trap of negative thinking and self-criticism. I'm committed to identifying the right problem."

Mastery Step

- Identify the right reason you are successful. Then discover what is really behind your challenges. HINT: It has nothing to do with NOT ENOUGH TIME.
- What are you doing well?
- What are you struggling with?
- Why are you able to do this well? Keep asking yourself "why?" until you get to the root answer.
- Why are you struggling? Keep asking yourself "why?" until you get to the root answer.
- What are you going to continue doing?
- What are you going to stop doing or change?

CHAPTER 9

Success in Action

Successful people are simply
those with successful habits.
— BRIAN TRACY

S uccess is staying on track for as long as possible – and getting back on track as quickly as possible.

This notion might be counterintuitive to chronic dieters whose eyes are set only on a "goal weight."

Before My Hungry Head, I defined my success by whether I had arrived at the promised land – my goal weight. I never gave much thought to how I would maintain that number. I didn't think about what I'd have to give up, either. I started feeling free from the diet prison when I came to understand what success was for me, when I should take action, and what actions I should take.

In Control

A fallacy of the diet mentality is that you'll hit "goal weight" and stay there. That's not how the human body works. It's normal for our body weight to fluctuate – even daily fluctuations happen as the amount of water in our body changes. It's not uncommon to see two- or three-pound weight losses OR gains that have nothing to do with real, lasting weight loss.

All too often, I see patients become anxious or discouraged based on these water shifts. Sometimes it's just enough discouragement to prompt the oh-what-the-hell eating plan. You know, the one where you might as well eat what you want because "the diet" isn't working anymore. This is the primary reason that I ask patients not to weigh themselves more than once a week. Why create unnecessary stress? If your weight goes up or down no more than two to three pounds, consider yourself a success. You're in control. Identify what you're doing well and keep doing it!

Take Action

On the other hand, take care not to fall into the over-confidence trap. This is when you see four- to five-pound weight increases but figure: "This ain't too bad. I'm still better than I was."

This seems to be the head-in-the-sand or wishful-thinking stage. Unless you have a medical condition causing large amounts of water retention, a four- to five-pound gain is probably a little water – and some fat. This is a sign to take some action. There's no need to panic. A few days of objective observation is probably enough to shed some light on the problem areas. Identifying and addressing underlying causes will get you back on track.

Time to Panic

Previous success at weight *loss* can provide a false sense of confidence. Who hasn't thought "I know I've put on *a few* pounds, but I'll be able to lose it again. I've done it before." This self-deception is often what lies between making real, lasting changes and a detour toward the latest diet-of-the-month. Even worse, enough time spent in this magical-thinking fog can result in seven-, eight- or 10-pound weight gain – or more. Now this is the time to panic!

You would think that this is when my phone rings most. But all too often, two- to three-pound water shifts cause more "panic" calls than gains of 10-plus pounds. Rather than reaching out, this seems to be the time when many people give up – or retreat with embarrassment.

There's no direct route to losing weight and keeping it off. Success is more than reaching a weight goal. It's the place where you can be healthy AND enjoy your life.

The process is much like the ebb and flow of the ocean tide. Sometimes it all goes well, and other times not so much. Ultimately, success starts with realistic goals and accepting that managing our weight is an ongoing process of applying six fundamental skills.

We've discussed them before, but let's go over them again:

1. **Objectively observing hunger, energy and cravings.** You need to become an alert observer, but don't get so caught up in collecting data that you don't make decisions.
3. **Analysis of your hunger cycle: determining when and what to eat.** Determine a pattern of what, when and where to eat that works best for you. Try to think of this in positive terms.
5. **Feeling your emotions, not eating them.** Allow yourself to feel the emotion and let it pass, like a wave on a beach. Don't get stuck in "drama."

7. **Retraining your brain with positive messages.** An excellent example: "That was good. I've had enough. I can have more later." But remember that you can't calm your brain unless you've fed and rested your body.

9. **Generating new ways of living between meals.** Make to-do lists that excite you rather than seeming like drudgery.

11. **Looking at the big picture to address the real problem,** not just the symptoms.

The most successful people I know have realistic goals and they apply each of these six skills at the right time. Those that struggle most tend to overuse one or two of these skills. For example, my most anxious patients tend to cycle between overanalyzing and feeling lots of emotions. Chronic dieters – trapped in the diet prison without realizing it – are often seduced by Pollyanna-like positivity and the hope that comes with starting something new. "This diet is different. This one's going to work – this time."

Practice these skills, and you'll get lasting weight loss. Sounds pretty easy? I suppose it might be if not for life's unknown, unplanned curve balls. No matter who you are, we are all susceptible to getting sick, leaving jobs, having kids, losing parents.

Dr. Anita Johnston, a clinical psychologist and expert on eating disorders, describes it well when she says, "Life is like an ocean. Things come in waves, some big ones, some little ones. But the waves never last. And there's always calm between the waves."

Johnston notes that the problem isn't the waves. It's that we don't know how to surf. She adds, "When we see a wave, most of us put the boogie board in front of our face. That's why the waves hurt so much."

My successful patients learned how to "surf." They learned to ride the ups and downs of life. They also created the right conditions for success. A closer look reveals that these patients have:

- Realistic goals.
- Access to food they enjoy.
- Fulfilling work or engaging activities.
- Physical movement they enjoy doing.
- People in their lives who support their lifestyle.
- Time to reflect on their personal achievements.

Do as much as you can alone. You can probably do more than you think. But there may be times or situations when you need more help.

You'll want to seek professional advice if you are on medications that contribute to weight gain. Weight-gaining medications include some anti-depressants and mood stabilizers, some diabetes medicines, corticosteroids, and anti-seizure drugs.

Other medications may cause chemical imbalance in the gut that leads to insatiable cravings. If you think your medications may be causing weight gain, consult your physician. DO NOT stop taking your medication without your doctor's consent.

There may be times when you're doing everything right and you're still gaining weight or unable to budge the scale. Again, talk to a professional health-care provider. You may have an underlying medical condition causing the stall. Some food sensitivities may cause extreme bloating that can be misconstrued as weight gain. Don't get discouraged. Get curious and talk with your physician.

When I was young, my dad would say, "Tell me who your friends are, and I'll tell you who you are." There's some evidence that friends can play a role in weight gain. If your social life is centered on eating out, meeting for drinks, or watching the game with beer and pizza, then you may find managing your weight more challenging than it would be if you were hanging around with active, outdoorsy types.

Keep in mind that it's nearly impossible to change your life without affecting those around you. Perhaps they will change, too. Maybe they won't. You may need to renegotiate some relationships if you want to stay on the success train.

Leah's Story

Leah, 46, is a perfect example of success in action. She is an empty-nester in the full swing of her career as a director for a large health-care organization. She is a very intelligent, well-educated professional who has battled her weight since childhood.

"All I can remember was being the smart, fat girl with glasses. Back then, it wasn't cool to be smart – or wear glasses. Forget about being fat. I tried to pretend the jokes didn't bother me, but they did. A lot."

Leah started dieting in her teens. By the time she was in college, she could teach just about any diet program – she understood nutrition well. Yet she still lost and regained more than 80 pounds multiple times before she opted to have gastric bypass surgery in 2003. At her highest weight, 305 pounds, Leah was suffering from severe degenerative hip disease. At age 32, weight-loss surgery would alleviate the pain and she would finally win the battle against her weight – or so she thought.

Initially, weight-loss surgery worked like magic. Leah lost 160 pounds within two years. A few foods that she used to eat made her feel sick, like ice cream and "one too many cookies," but otherwise, she could eat almost anything. She was working full time as a nurse and picked up a few extra shifts every week to make some extra money.

"I didn't know what to do with myself. I figured working another job might fill the void. Anyway, the money helped pay off all the shopping I was doing after surgery."

Five years had passed since Leah's weight-loss surgery when her lucky break came. A new health-care organization in the city recruited her for a management position. It was an opportunity for which she was waiting.

"I was so happy. I was excited to have the responsibility, the title, the money. I never would have gotten this far if I was still 280 pounds."

Leah took the job, even though it would require a two-hour commute to and from work. The long hours in the office were tiring. And the commute was unbearable.

"I could barely stay awake. My mornings consisted of drive-through coffees. On the way home, I would munch on candy in the car just to stay awake. I'd just crash as soon as I walked in the door."

She was up 54 "effing" pounds. "It didn't get worse than this. Weight-loss surgery was my last resort."

After taking a big step back, Leah could see that food wasn't the real problem. Nor was it her weight. She wanted more out of life – something she couldn't find in a mall or nightclub.

Leah made some big decisions. She took a job for less money that was closer to home. A hard look at life between meals helped her identify her true passion – she wants to help others. She enjoyed running, but it was time-consuming and lonely.

She joined a running group after the Boston marathon bombing to raise money for the bombing victims. She had purpose now – she was running for a reason. She was part of something bigger than herself. "I'm actually feeling athletic. I feel like I belong."

Running is more than a way to manage weight. Leah made it a lifestyle. She learned to eat better and train better. She lost all the weight she re-gained and then some. Added lean muscle. And, more important, a sense of accomplishment.

Leah was promoted to a position higher than the job she had left. The money is great – and she's building her savings. "I feel like I don't need to shop all the time – well, at least as much. I love what I'm doing now. I love the people I'm with. It's not perfect, but it's damn close!"

CHAPTER 10

Sailing

I am not afraid of storms
for I am learning to sail my ship.
— LOUISA MAY ALCOTT

didn't realize sailing was so tough until I tried it.

I was on a 24-foot open sailboat. No inboard motor. No kicker. Just a sail. Getting my boat from point A to point B required a series of exercises that were all weather-dependent. Not fun for someone who loves to be in complete control! A firm grip on the tiller kept the boat pointed in the right direction. I adjusted my speed by hauling in the mainsheet when the wind was too strong and changing tack when the wind pushed me off course. Other times, I had to adjust my own expectations when the wind unexpectedly died down.

Damn. Sailing was just like my life. And a lot like weight control.

You can't just jump on a diet plan and expect to sail on to success. It was only when I accepted this – and I mean accepted it, deep in my core – did the process of managing my weight become easier. This acceptance allowed me to break the chronic cycle of naively buying into quick-fix weight-loss schemes and suffering the pain of rebound pounds. My patients who continually do well don't expect easy results. They know that managing their weight is a process. They've accepted that it's something they have to do daily – one day at a time.

There's no direct route to everlasting weight loss. For me, it's been more like a meandering journey. Progress required a real understanding of my body, my life goals and what I was willing to give up to achieve them. Was it really just weight loss? Or controlling my cravings? Or was it something bigger?

Along my travels, I've learned to listen to my hunger. My physical hunger. My emotional hunger. And my spiritual hunger. They each have a voice. And they each want to be heard, understood, and satisfied. Although there's no GPS route with turn-by-turn instructions, each step of the My Hungry Head program helped me chart a direction that makes sense for my life.

It's no secret that you can achieve weight loss with or without surgery. Heck, I've met patients who have lost more than 100 pounds up to 16 times!

Ava, 65, a non-surgical weight-loss patient did just that. She suffered from a soul-destroying legacy of dieting that spanned more than five decades. Keeping weight off has been the ongoing challenge for surgical and non-surgical weight-loss programs across the nation.

Currently, less than 20 percent of surgical weight-loss patients follow up with their programs after two years, and even fewer follow up after three years. I've met far too many patients who shared their embarrassment to return to their doctors because they have regained much of their weight. Big-box commercial programs rely on the 80 percent who regain weight to purchase another round of their program.

Sharing the Journey

It sucks to sail alone.

We've all heard stories about the person who sailed around the world – all alone. Some people find peace in long stretches of solitude. The vast majority of us don't.

Humans are social animals. We learn from each other. We flourish with support. I found that sailing with others is fun. It made the journey less scary for me. But sailing with others is different from having a party on shore. I still have to do the work. Pay attention. Know where I'm going. Make decisions. There's nothing static about sailing – or managing weight. But somehow, sharing the journey with others often seems to ease the way.

At first I was afraid to sail – I feared the worst. My real fear was the ocean. Just the thought of its vast, powerful force overwhelms me. It's the same feeling I can get when I think about the processed-food industry, advertising, the media, and the ever-present social pressures to be thin, young and beautiful ... all of it can make me feel like a tiny boat being tossed like a toy in the omnipotent sea.

Learning the ins and outs of a sailboat, how to read a chart, and when to maneuver the sails lessened my anxiety. I had a great teacher. He broke it all down in a way that made sense to me. He understood my anxiety. I learned critical, yet comforting, lessons from him, such as knowing when to go sailing – and when to stay home. How to locate a shelter – and when to pull in to a safe harbor.

My Hungry Head is a process. It's way of being – kind of like sailing. I don't have to sail alone. I don't have to manage my weight alone. And neither do you.

Helpful Resources

My Hungry Head.com

Whether you plan to have weight-loss surgery, are in need of post-surgical guidance, or want to control weight on your own, My Hungry Head provides the direction you need to achieve results. My Hungry Head was developed to help individuals control their weight and feel better about their bodies through education, integration, and transformation of a healthier lifestyle. My Hungry Head is NOT the diet regimen or exercise routine that you've already tried. Our mission is to educate patients on the emotional, physiological and sociological triggers that stimulate hunger so that they can better control their appetites and can make positive changes that lead to long-term weight loss. Contact www.myhungryhead.com to enroll in one of our online programs, live courses or weekend retreats.

My Hungry Head Certification Program

We encourage clinicians to become certified to offer My Hungry Head through their own practices or medical facilities. Our professional services team teaches you how to administer and manage the program, and offer it directly to your patients, live or online. We provide all of the resources required to get the program up and running quickly. Contact info@myhungryhead.com to learn more.

Finding North Collaborative

In many ancient cultures, *north* represents illumination, discovery and understanding. The Finding North Collaborative uses these principles to help individuals, groups, and organizations listen to their intuition and find their internal compass. By abiding by these principles, participants create a healthier lifestyle, develop creativity, and find resilience and inspiration to solve ongoing challenges of personal and professional life. To learn more, contact Finding North Collaborative at info@findingnorthcollaborative.com.

Light of the Moon Café.com

This is an online space where women of all ages from around the world can gather to be embraced in the warmth of a women's circle and have experiences that nourish the deepest, most intimate parts of their being. Anita Johnston, a psychologist/storyteller, and Elisabeth Peterson, a dietitian/group leader, have worked many years in the field of disordered eating. They are passionate about using women's circles for healing struggles with food, eating and weight. Contact www.myhungryhead.com for a program discount.

Livliga™ Portioned Controlled Dinnerware

Livliga offers our favorite portion-controlled dinnerware. Its simply elegant, intelligent designs are created to subtly guide you in eating a balanced meal with appropriate serving sizes. Your mind and body look for external cues to tell you how much to eat. Food served on beautifully designed, right-sized dishware looks plentiful and appealing, sending positive signals to your brain, leaving you feeling nourished and satisfied. Livliga calls these VisualQs.

We agree that it is possible to be mindful of what you eat and fully enjoy your meal and the process of eating. Eating food from right-sized dishware that is also thoughtfully and beautifully designed is a key element to success and satisfaction. www.livliga.com

BeSoul Dance™

BeSoul Dance provides an opportunity to connect to your deepest self through movement and self-expression. Choreography is simple and enlivening, music is fantastic and varied, we dance together to get fit in body, mind and soul. BeSoul Dance is available to all body and fitness types. Certification Programs are also available for movement instructors. For more information, contact www.yogaandniaforlife.com

Intuition Nutrition

Provides coaching and consulting in traditional weight loss and nutrition before and after weight-loss surgery. Clinician Elizabeth Dahlgren approaches nutrition in a whole body, personalized way. With evidence-based advice, she provides the tools to make food and lifestyle decisions that will properly fuel your body. In addition to supporting the My Hungry Head process, Intuition Nutrition promotes mindfulness and body awareness and values its impact on your wellness. www.intuitionnutritionllc.com

Weight Loss Surgery & Beyond (WLS&B)

Founded by Paul and Heather Vargas, this far-reaching support group knows weight management is not all rainbows. In this well-run, closed Facebook group, surgical weight-loss patients are "real", respectful and honest. They laugh together, they learn and fail together, and they inspire each other daily. WLS&B is also a very welcoming group for post-op veterans who may have fallen off-track and need an understanding venue to re-establish connection and accountability. Key to the health of this group is its hard-working administrative team, which ensures daily engagement and appropriate communication between members.

Obesity Action Coalition (OAC)

The Obesity Action Coalition is a more than 50,000 member-strong 501(c)(3) national nonprofit organization dedicated to giving a voice to the individual affected by the disease of obesity and helping individuals along their journey toward better health through education, advocacy and support. Our core focuses are to raise awareness and improve access to the prevention and treatment of obesity, provide evidence-based education on obesity and its treatments, fight to eliminate weight bias and discrimination, elevate the conversation on weight and its impact on health, and offer a community of support for the individual affected. www.obesityaction.org

Binge Eating Disorder Association (BEDA)

Founded in 2008, the Binge Eating Disorder Association is a national organization focused on providing leadership, recognition, prevention, and treatment of BED and associated weight stigma. Through outreach, education and advocacy, BEDA facilitates increased awareness, proper diagnosis and treatment of BED.

BEDA promotes excellence in care for those who live with, and those who treat, binge eating disorder and its associated conditions. BEDA is committed to promoting cultural acceptance of, and respect for, the natural diversity of sizes, as well as promoting a goal of improved health, which may or may not include weight change. bedaonline.org

National Association of Men with Eating Disorders (NAMED)

NAMED is the only organization in the United States exclusively dedicated to representing and providing support to males with eating disorders. Historically, boys and men with eating disorders have received inadequate attention, research, support, and intervention. NAMED plays a vital role in filling this gap by offering support, as well as information and resources, to this underrepresented population and their families and by serving as a clearinghouse for treatment providers and researchers. www.namedinc.org

National Eating Disorder Association (NEDA)

The National Eating Disorders Association (NEDA) is the leading 501(c)(3) nonprofit organization in the United States advocating on behalf of and supporting individuals and families affected by eating disorders. Reaching millions every year, the organization campaigns for prevention, improved access to quality treatment, and increased research funding to better understand and treat eating disorders. It works with partners and volunteers to develop programs and tools to help everyone who seeks assistance. www.nationaleatingdisorders.org

Obesity Medicine Association

We strive to provide the best resources for our members to help them advance the field of obesity medicine, deliver evidence-based treatments, and improve the lives of patients affected by obesity. We offer unique, accredited educational opportunities and promote the sharing of information among our members to enrich the learning experience. We support advocacy efforts through our involvement in the Obesity Care Continuum and the American Medical Association House of Delegates.

We host educational events for health-care providers with a wide range of expertise, from those just starting out in obesity medicine to those who practice obesity medicine full time. Our education focuses on the comprehensive treatment approach – nutrition, physical activity, behavior and medication – and providing optimal care for patients affected by obesity. www.obesitymedicine.org

American Society of Metabolic & Bariatric Surgery (ASMBS)

The vision of the society is to improve public health and well-being by lessening the burden of the disease of obesity and related diseases throughout the world.

Founded in 1983, foremost U.S. surgeons have formed the society's leadership and have established an excellent organization with educational and support programs for surgeons and integrated health professionals. The purpose of the society is to advance the art and science of metabolic and bariatric surgery by continually improving the quality and safety of care and treatment of people with obesity and related diseases. www.asmbs.org

References

Chapter 3: The Objective Observer

James McBride. <u>The Color of Water: A Black Man's Tribute to His White Mother</u>. New York: Riverhead Books, 1996.

http://articles.chicagotribune.com/1994-04-05/features/9404050022_1_
eat-smart-first-book-specialty-book

Chapter 4: Your Hunger Cycle

Ahmed, QA. "Metabolic Complications of Obstructive Sleep Apnea Syndrome." <u>The American Journal of the Medical Sciences</u> (2008).

Karamanakos, Stavros N., V. Konstantinos, F. Kalfarentzos, T. Alexandrides. "Weight Loss, Appetite Suppression, and Changes in Fasting and Postprandial Ghrelin and Peptide-YY Levels After Roux-en-Y Gastric Bypass and Sleeve Gastrectomy: A Prospective, Double Blind Study." <u>Annals of Surgery</u>. 247 (2008): 401-407.

Le Roux, Carel, et al. (2007) "Gut Hormones as Mediators of Appetite and Weight Loss After Roux-en-Y Gastric Bypass." Annals of Surgery. 246 (2007): 780-785.

McMinn, Julie E., D. Sindelar, P. Havel, M. Schwartz. "Leptin Deficiency Induced by Fasting Impairs the Satiety Response to Cholecystokinin." Endocrinology. 141 (2011).

Morton, Gregory J., D. Baskin, M. Schwartz. "Leptin Action in the Forebrain Regulates the Hindbrain Response to Satiety Signals." Journal of Clinical Investigation. 115 (2005): 703-710.

Moss, Michael. Salt, Sugar, Fat: How the Food Giants Hooked Us. New York: Random House, 2013.

Sahu, A., "Resistance to the Satiety Action of Leptin Following Chronic Central Leptin Infusion is Associated with the Development of Leptin Resistance in Neuropeptide Y Neurones." Journal of Neuroendocrinology. 14 (2002): 796-804.

Spiegel K, Tasali E, Penev P, Cauter E. "Brief Communication: Sleep Curtailment in Healthy Young Men Is Associated with Decreased Leptin Levels, Elevated Ghrelin Levels, and Increased Hunger and Appetite." Annals of Internal Medicine. 141 (2004): 846-850.

Chapter 6: Retrain Your Brain

http://psychology.about.com/od/historyofpsychology/f/father-of-psychology.htm

Chapter 7: Living Between Meals

Campbell, Joseph and Bill Moyers. The Power of Myth. New York: Doubleday, 1988.

Selhub, Eva M. and Alan C. Logan. Your Brain On Nature:

The Science of Nature's Influence on Your Health, Happiness and Vitality. John Wiley & Sons, 2012.

Young, S. N. "How to Increase Serotonin in the Human

Brain Without Drugs." Journal of Psychiatry & Neuroscience. 32 (2007): 394–399.

Sprouse-Blum, A. S., Smith, G., Sugai, D., & Parsa, F. D. "Understanding Endorphins and Their Importance in Pain Management." Hawaii Medical Journal. 69 (2010): 70–71.

Berk, Lee S. and Stanley A. Tan. [beta] "Endorphin and HGH Increase Are Associated with Both the Anticipation and Experience of Mirthful Laughter." The FASEB Journal. 20 (2006): A382

Barraza, Jorge A. and Paul J. Zak. "Empathy Toward Strangers Triggers Oxytocin Release and Subsequent Generosity." (2009) DOI: 10.1111/j.17496632.2009.04504.x

Odendaal, J.S.J. (2000) "Animal-Assisted Therapy — Magic or Medicine?" Journal of Psychosomatic Research. 49 (2000): 275-280.

Bernstein, Marcus, D. A., C. D., Constantin, J. M., Kunkel, F. A., Breuer, P. and Hanlon, R. B. "Impact of Animal-Assisted Therapy for Outpatients with Fibromyalgia." Pain Medicine. 14 (2013): 43–51.

Moreira, F. A. and Lutz, B. "The Endocannabinoid System: Emotion, Learning and Addiction." Addiction Biology. 13 (2008): 196–212.

Salimpoor, Valorie N, et al. "Anatomically Distinct Dopamine Release During Anticipation and Experience of Peak Emotion to Music. Nature Neuroscience. 14 (2011): 257–262.

Chapter 9: Success in Action

Higa, Kelvin, et al. (2009) Laparoscopic Roux-en-Y Gastric Bypass: 10-Year Follow-Up. Surgery for Obesity and Related Diseases. 7 (2009): 516-525.

Puzziferri N, Roshek TB, III, Mayo HG, Gallagher R, Belle SH, Livingston EH. "Long-Term Follow-up After Bariatric Surgery: A Systematic Review." JAMA. 312 (2014): 934-942.

About the Authors

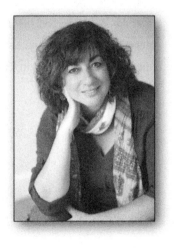

arybeth Sherrin is a licensed behavioral therapist specializing in obesity and binge eating. She has worked with more than 7,000 patients, helping them develop effective strategies to maintain weight loss. She is also the executive director of the Institute for Bariatric Education, where she directs the development of educational, support and community programs for surgical and non-surgical weight-loss patients. Sherrin has a master's degree in counseling psychology from the University of Massachusetts/ Boston and a master's degree in psychology from Harvard University. She lives in the Boston area with her husband and two boys.

Maria Skinner is a leading body movement expert and the creator of movement and body appreciation programs. She specializes in helping patients struggling with weight and body image following significant weight loss. Skinner is the creator of Move My Way™ and BeSoul™, a Huffington Post contributor, and a former black-belt Nia technique instructor, teacher-trainer, and faculty member. She has a bachelor of arts degree from NYU. Maria has a studio and private practice in Concord, Massachusetts.

Paul Jablow is a journalist with nearly four decades of experience in the newspaper business, including 30 years as a reporter and editor at The Philadelphia Inquirer. He has written and edited for freelance clients, including the Robert Wood Johnson Foundation and Children's Hospital of Philadelphia. His most recent collaboration was with Dr. Thomas N. Tavantzis on the book *Hardwired*. A native of New York City, Jablow lives in Bryn Mawr, Pennsylvania.

Notes

Notes

Notes

Notes

Notes

Notes

Notes

Notes

Notes

Notes

Notes

Notes

Notes

Notes

43770526R00114